NEUROLOGY - LABORATORY AND CLINICAL RESEARCH DEVELOPMENTS

SEIZURES AND ANTI-EPILEPTIC DRUGS

NEUROLOGY - LABORATORY AND CLINICAL RESEARCH DEVELOPMENTS

Additional books in this series can be found on Nova's website under the Series tab.

Additional E-books in this series can be found on Nova's website under the E-book tab.

NEUROLOGY - LABORATORY AND CLINICAL RESEARCH DEVELOPMENTS

SEIZURES AND ANTI-EPILEPTIC DRUGS

WILLARD HOSTEN
AND
ALEPH BURTSEV
EDITORS

Nova Science Publishers, Inc.
New York

For permission to use material from this book please contact us:
Telephone 631-231-7269; Fax 631-231-8175
Web Site: http://www.novapublishers.com

Additional color graphics may be available in the e-book version of this book.

Library of Congress Cataloging-in-Publication Data

Seizures and anti-epileptic drugs / editors, Willard Hosten and Aleph Burtsev.
p. ; cm.
Includes bibliographical references and index.
ISBN 978-1-62100-255-0 (hardcover)
I. Hosten, Willard. II. Burtsev, Aleph.
[DNLM: 1. Epilepsy--drug therapy. 2. Anticonvulsants--therapeutic use. WL 385]
LC classification not assigned
616.8'53061--dc23

2011032416

Published by Nova Science Publishers, Inc. † New York

Contents

Preface

This book presents current research in the study of the prevention, recognition and treatment of seizures and the use of anti-epileptic drugs. Topics discussed in this compilation include the behavioral comorbidities in adult patients with epilepsy; seizure control and behavioral and cognitive outcomes in patients taking anti-epileptic drugs; epilepsy related injuries; the clinical pharmacokinetic characteristics of novel antiepileptic drugs; familial cortical myoclonic tremor with epilepsy; panayiotopoulos syndrome and psychosocial consequences for people living with seizures.

Chapter I - Epilepsy is a common health problem. Seizures are only one aspect of epilepsy. Patients with epilepsy have a high prevalence of inter-ictal psychiatric comorbid disorders. Common behavioral/emotional syndromes which are seen frequently in epileptic patients include depression, anxiety, psychosis, attention-deficit, obsessive compulsive and personality disorders, aggression and suicide. The mechanisms of psychiatric comorbidity with epilepsy are poorly understood. An increasing body of literature points to a complex relationship between psychiatric and seizure disorders. In fact, organic as well as social variables are contributed. A shared pathophysiological mechanism, neuronal plasticity and impairment of cellular metabolism associated with the process of epileptogenesis as well as genetic, psychosocial and iatrogenic factors are fundamental determinants. The potential for antiepileptic drugs (AEDs) to adversely impact behavior is of significant concern as they are the major therapeutic modality for control of seizures. Even their modest effects canbe of clinical significant and affect the patient's qualityof life. AEDs have both negative and positive psychotropic effects. AEDs are able to improve behavior because of their anti-seizure, neurotransmitters' modulation and psychotrophic effects. However, increasing GABAergic inhibitory activity, glutamate blockage activity and alteration of serotoninergic, adrenergic and noradrenergic neurotrasmitters and pathways might contribute to behavioral changes associated with AEDs. The progress in recognition of psychiatric comorbidities related to epilepsy and their pathophysiologic mechanisms should move the treatment of patients towards a comprehensive biopsychosocial model that focuses on the whole person rather than simply on the disease process.

Chapter II - Anti-epileptic drugs (AEDs) are characterized by a variety of mechanisms of action, leading to different anticonvulsant activities and behavioral/psychotropic profiles. At the one end of the pharmacodynamic spectrum are AEDs potentiating inhibitory gamma-aminobutyric acid (GABA) neurotransmission. The other end of the spectrum comprises

AEDs attenuating excitatory glutamate neurotransmission. GABA-enhancing AEDs have sedating and anti-manic effects, while the second group is characterized by antidepressant effects. This chapter reviews the mechanisms of action, main clinical indications, and behavioral and cognitive profiles of a range of AEDs. In clinical practice, both patients' characteristics and AEDs' cognitive and behavioral profiles should be taken into account in order to maximize benefits in terms of seizure control and behavioral and cognitive outcome.

Chapter III - Since 1960 there have been reports that those with epilepsy are more prone to injuries compared to those without epilepsy. The largest population-based study to date reported that persons with epilepsy were 1.4 times more likely to have sustained an injury for which medical attention was sought. Risk factors for injuries have been reported to include seizure frequency, disease duration, treatment duration, cognitive handicap and seizure-type. Most of the seizure-types included in studies were tonic-clonic seizures and seizures causing falls. Seizures resulting in falls increase the risk of concussion and other injuries. Most recurrent seizure-related injuries involve head injury. Most injuries are minor. However more serious injury rates are increased. The risk of fracture is elevated almost 2-fold, either resulting directly from seizure-induced injury or predisposed by drug-induced reduction in bone mineral density. Hip and femur fractures are the most common. Submersion injury has a high mortality; the risk of submersion in people with epilepsy is 18.7 fold higher than in the general population. Although population and prospective studies have reported no significant difference in burns between persons with epilepsy and those without, there are conflicting data. The risk of motor vehicle accidents in drivers with epilepsy also appears increased, albeit marginally. While it is appropriate to mandate appropriate restrictions to reduce injury, such as limitations on driving and certain sports or activities, excessive limitations may further limit achievement of independence. Appropriate vitamin D and calcium supplementation and periodic measurement of bone mineral density in those at risk for osteoporosis are recommended.

Chapter IV - The choice of an antiepileptic drug (AED) is usually based upon the epileptic seizure type. However, pharmacokinetic (PK) characteristics of AEDs may be valuable support in choosing the optimal therapeutic option for the individual patient. The novel (second and third generation) AEDs include: eslicarbazepine acetate, felbamate, gabapentin, lacosamide, lamotrigine, levetiracetam, oxcarbazepine, pregabalin, rufinamide, stiripentol, tiagabine, topiramate, vigabatrin, and zonisamide. Although, these drugs belong to the same group, their individual PK characteristics differ. Gabapentin, unlike other new AEDs, is characterised by dose-dependent absorption, which is presumably caused by saturable L-amino acid transport system, and therefore its bioavailability ranges from 35-60%. Furthermore, gabapentin, pregabalin and vigabatrin are eliminated completely, while levetiracetam and topiramate are eliminated predominantly through the renal system. Therefore, PK variability of these individual drugs is less pronounced and more predictable in comparison to older AEDs. Their potential for drug interactions is minor, and consequently they have major clinical importance for patients with impaired hepatic function. On the other hand, felbamate, lamotrigine, oxcarbazepine, tiagabine and zonisamide are eliminated via metabolic pathways, either cytochrome P (CYP) 450, or conjugation dependent transformation. Oxcarbazepine is a prodrug, and its active metabolite is licarbazepine. These drugs interact with other drugs, and disease conditions, which alter the activity of metabolic enzymes; thus these changes in PK commonly have clinical implications. Gabapentin, levetiracetam and tiagabine do not induce or inhibit hepatic metabolism enzymes. Felbamate demonstrated an inducing effect on CYP 3A4 isoenzyme, and inhibition effect on CYP 2C19 and on β-oxidation of valproic acid. Lamotrigine induces its own metabolism, and some reports imply a decrease of valproic acid levels during concomitant treatment with lamotrigine. Oxcarbazepine induces CYP 3A4, 3A5, and uridine diphosphate glucuronyl transfereases (UGT), and inhibits the metabolism of phenytoin via CYP 2C19 isoenzyme. Similar induction and inhibition characteristics are attributed to topiramate, while some studies indicate that zonisamide may have inhibition potential on phenytoin metabolism. In general, novel AEDs have linear PK, low plasma protein binding, and renal elimination, so their PK is more favorable in comparison with carbamazepine, phenobarbitone and valproic acid. This chapter gives a review of PK parameters of novel AEDs and its' variability based on age, comorbidities, concomitant therapy, and highlights the need of therapeutic drug monitoring.

Chapter V - The association between tremor and epileptic seizures was firstly reported 36 years ago. In 1990, sporadic cases tremor with a cortical origin consisting of irregular, distal twitches of the extremities associated with seizures were named as cortical tremor. Subsequently, familial cases of cortical tremor, myoclonus and epileptic seizures, representing autosomal dominant inheritance were described under several names, such as familial adult myoclonic epilepsy (FAME), benign adult familial myoclonic epilepsy (BAFME), autosomal dominant cortical myoclonus and epilepsy (ADCME). Recently, all of these syndromes were considered as one phenotype and proposed the term "familial cortical myoclonic tremor with epilepsy" (FCMTE). In briefly, FCMTE is an autosomal dominant disorder characterized by adult onset cortical tremor, myoclonus and seizures. The clinical features of FCMTE include involuntary rhythmic myoclonic movements (tremor) of the distal extremities, usually fingers movements, generalized tonic-clonic seizures (GTCS), and mental retardation. EEG shows generalized and focal spike and wave complexes. Somatosensory evoked potentials (SEP) indicated enlarged cortical components and enhanced long-loop reflex I (LLRI). Neuroimaging is usually normal although nonspecific abnormalities are sometimes reported in patients with mental retardation, such as mild enlargement of the subarachnoid spaces or of the lateral ventricles. Antiepileptic drugs, including phenobarbital, valproic acid, benzodiazepines, are effective to this syndrome. Three loci have been identified on chromesome 8q23.3-q24.11, 2p11.1-q12.2 and 5p15.31-p15.

Chapter VI - Epilepsy is the commonest serious neurological disorder worldwide. Despite multiple antiepileptic drug (AED) options, it has been established that 20-30% of epilepsies are not controlled by antiepileptic drugs. Drug resistance in epilepsy thus becomes an important clinical problem. The current developments in molecular medicine have led to the perspective that individual differences in responsiveness to drugs of various pharmacological classes, like many other human traits, are the result of a complex combination of genetic and environmental factors. According to this perspective, genes not only predispose to epilepsy but also determine responsiveness to antiepileptic drugs. Genetic variations of genes can potentially affect individual responsiveness to the drug at several steps that include drug absorption, drug distribution, drug metabolism, elimination and drug concentration at target sites. The metabolism of drug greatly influences its concentration in blood and target organ. The polymorphisms in the genes involved in drug metabolizing enzymes determine the drug levels in the plasma, thus affecting the effective dose and toxicity for antiepileptic drug. Some forms of idiopathic epilepsy have been found to be due to mutations in ion channels. There are also evidences of link between channel abnormalities and drug responsiveness in epilepsy.

Several studies have documented association between drug transporter protein (MDR1 or ABCB1) genetic variants with drug resistance in epilepsy. Therefore, polymorphic genetic variants of drug metabolizing enzymes, multi drug transporters, receptors and ion channels are prime candidates for studies of drug responsiveness and adverse drug reaction in epilepsy. In conclusion, new developments in pharmacogenomics hold great promise of antiepileptic drugs matched to specific genotypes.

Chapter VII - Panayiotopoulos Syndrome is one of the benign childhood seizure susceptibility syndromes, which has drawn increasing attention in the last decade. Panayiotopoulos Syndrome is common, affecting around 6% of children with afebrile seizures, manifests as autonomic seizures and autonomic status epilepticus that are specific to childhood, provides links with mainly rolandic epilepsy, and is frequently misdiagnosed as encephalitis and other nonepileptic disorders. Interictal EEG shows in 80% of patients multifocal spikes with occipital predominance often shifting from one region to another in sequential EEG recordings of the same patient. Prognosis with respect to seizure remission and neuropsychological development is excellent. Continuous treatment with antiepileptic drugs is usually not needed. This review focuses on the clinical and electroencephalographic features of Panayiotopoulos Syndrome with particular emphasis on genetic and neurobehavioral aspects.

Chapter VIII - Epilepsy affects different domains of an individual's life: in addition to health, independence, education and employment are all tainted. Beyond seizures, changes in mental health, behavioral alterations and variable cognitive function are central to epilepsy. Several studies have explored the relationship between behavioral impairment and seizure-related variables. In more recent years, particular emphasis has been placed on the clinical challenge presented by anti-epileptic drugs (AEDs). AEDs have various mechanisms of action and therefore generate a wide and diverse spectrum of anti-convulsant, psychiatric, and adverse effect profiles. AEDs may be presented in two classes, divided according to predominant psychotropic profile. The first group consists of valproate, gabapentin, tiagabine and vigabatrin. This cluster is characterized by potentiation of gamma-aminobutyric acid inhibitory neurotransmission. Resultant effects include cognitive slowing, anxiolytic as well anti-manic effects. Conversely, a second cluster is defined by predominantly glutamate excitatory neurotransmission. This cluster includes lamotrigine and felbamate, and is associated with activating and anti-depressant effects. In accordance with this dual classification system, the present chapter provides a detailed description of the behavioral profile of the newer AEDs. Additionally, a brief discussion on aspects such as clinical indications, pharmacology, toxicology, efficacy and tolerability is included. It is essential that AEDs therapy offers an acceptable balance between optimum seizure control and minimal disturbance to behavior and cognition.

Chapter IX - The consequences that seizures may have on a patient's psychological and social well-being are often underestimated. People with epilepsy have much higher rates of co-morbid depression, as well as suicide, compared with the background population. Screening for depressive symptoms, as well appropriate treatment and referral, is an essential part in the management of the patient with seizures. Although a person living with epilepsy may only spend a few minutes each year in seizure, it is the unpredictability of the next event that may necessitate lifestyle changes. It is important, however, to balance the risks of subsequent seizures with the psychosocial implications of placing restrictions on the patient's work and lifestyle. This chapter focuses on how the treating clinician addresses the psychological and social implication for people who live with seizures. Specific attention is paid towards co-morbid depression and suicide, as well as stigma associated with epilepsy, and the vocational and lifestyle implications of having seizures.

Chapter X - Pharmacokinetics of antiepileptic drugs (AED's) and oral contraceptives (OC's) can interact bi-directionally. AED's have a potential influence on the effect of OC's and pose thereby a risk of un-intended pregnancy as well as OC's may decrease the effect of some AED's and increase the risk of seizure deterioration. The consequences are of major concern. Contraceptive failure may be disastrous for most women but is critical for women who are taking AED's because of the teratogenetic potential of the AED's. In addition, AED failure can seriously influence on many psychosocial aspects of the patient's life. The magnitude of the drug-drug interactions shows in general wide inter-individual variability and the change in the elimination rate is often unpredictable and can be influenced by a number of co-variants. Change in OC use should therefore be assisted by AED monitoring and adequate dose adjustment whenever possible and AED's without pharmacokinetic interaction potentials may be considered as drug of first choices for women who use OC's.

In: Seizures and Anti-Epileptic Drugs
Editors: Willard Hosten and Aleph Burtsev

ISBN: 978-1-62100-255-0

Chapter I

Behavioral Comorbidities in Adult Patients with Epilepsy: Special Emphasis to Antiepileptic Medications

Sherifa A. Hamed*
Department of Neurology and Psychiatry,
Assiut University Hospital, Assiut, Egypt

Abstract

Epilepsy is a common health problem. Seizures are only one aspect of epilepsy. Patients with epilepsy have a high prevalence of inter-ictal psychiatric comorbid disorders. Common behavioral/emotional syndromes which are seen frequently in epileptic patients include depression, anxiety, psychosis, attention-deficit, obsessive compulsive and personality disorders, aggression and suicide. The mechanisms of psychiatric comorbidity with epilepsy are poorly understood. An increasing body of literature points to a complex relationship between psychiatric and seizure disorders. In fact, organic as well as social variables are contributed. A shared pathophysiological mechanism, neuronal plasticity and impairment of cellular metabolism associated with the process of epileptogenesis as well as genetic, psychosocial and iatrogenic factors are fundamental determinants. The potential for antiepileptic drugs (AEDs) to adversely impact behavior is of significant concern as they are the major therapeutic modality for control of seizures. Even their modest effects canbe of clinical significant and affect the patient's qualityof life. AEDs have both negative and positive psychotropic effects. AEDs are able to improve behavior because of their anti-seizure, neurotransmitters' modulation and psychotrophic effects. However, increasing GABAergic inhibitory activity, glutamate blockage activity and alteration of serotoninergic, adrenergic and

* Corresponding author: Sherifa Ahmad Hamed, MBBch, MSc., M.D. Consultant Neurologist. Associate Professor, Department of Neurology and Psychiatry, Assiut University Hospital, Assiut, Egypt. P.O.Box 71516; Telephone: +2 088 2374904; Fax:: +2 088 2333327;+2 088 2332278; Email: hamed_sherifa@yahoo.com

noradrenergic neurotrasmitters and pathways might contribute to behavioral changes associated with AEDs. The progress in recognition of psychiatric comorbidities related to epilepsy and their pathophysiologic mechanisms should move the treatment of patients towards a comprehensive biopsychosocial model that focuses on the whole person rather than simply on the disease process.

Keywords: Epilepsy; anti-epileptic drugs; behavioral/emotional or psychiatric comorbidities; neurotransmitters, psychosocial variables, biopsychosocial approach

Abbreviations

(TLE)	Temporal lobe epilepsy
(HS)	Hippocampal sclerosis
(AEDs)	Antiepileptic drugs
(OCD)	Obsessvive compulsive disorder
(ADHD)	Attention deficit hyperactivity disorder
(PIP)	Postictal psychosis
(PB)	Phenobarbital
(VGB)	Vigabatrin
(TPM)	Topiramate
(ZNC)	Zonisamide
(TGB)	Tiagabin
(LEV)	Levitracetam
(FBM)	Felbamate
(PHT)	Phenytoin
(CBZ)	Carbamazepine
(OXC)	Oxcarbazepine
(GBP)	Gabapentin
(VPA)	Valproate
(LTG)	Lamotrigine
(PGB)	Pregabalin
(ETX)	ethosuximide
(TCAs)	Tricyclic antidepressants

A. Introduction

Epilepsy is one of the most important and common chronic medical problems. The prevalence of epilepsy in general population is ~8.2 per 1,000 [1]. It is higher in developing countries (as in Colombia, Ecuador, Egypt, India, Liberia, Nigeria, Panama, United Republic of Tanzania and Venezuela) in which a prevalence of 10-12.9 per 1,000 were reported [2,3]. Fortunately, ~65% of patients with epilepsy become seizure free within few years (1-2 years). In the remaining (~25-35%) seizures are resistant to treatment with currently available AEDs. Hippocampal damage (hippocampal sclerosis or HS) was observed in 60–70% of medically intractable patients with epilepsy exposed to hippocampal lobectomy surgery [4]. The hippocampus and related area has been implicated in seizure-induced behavioral and cognitive disorders.

While epilepsy is defined by the presence of recurrent seizures due to sudden electrical misfiring of neurons or nerve cells in the epileptic's brain, it is complicated by a high rate of behavioral or psychiatric comorbid symptomatologies and disorders. Behavioral symptomatologies associated with epilepsy may occur peri-ictally (pre-ictal, ictal and post-ictal), and inter-ictally. Peri-ictal behavioral symptomatologies do not usually require treatment as improvement in seizure frequency is expected to reduce their occurrence [5-8].Inter-ictal behavioral symptomatologies are frequently mild and reversible, however, some patients with interactable epilepsy have enduring behavioral symptoms or disorder that require aggressive treatment. The common inter-ictal behavioral disorders include: depression, anxiety, psychosis, obcessive-compulsive, attention-deficit, personality disorders, aggression and suicide [9-17].

The inter-ictal psychiatric comorbidities seen with epilepsy have been found to be correlated with number of variables including psychosocial variables (as stigma, learning problems, unemployment, inability to obtain a driving licence) [18,19], demographic-, clinical- and epilepsy- related variables (as age, gender, age at onset, type of seizures, site and side of structural brain lesion, seizure frequency and duration of epilepsy) [20-23], and treatment-related variables (iatrogenic) or adverse effects from antiepileptic medications [24-26]. In fact, the mechanisms of psychiatric comorbidity with epilepsy are complex and poorly understood.

Functional (psychosocial), structural (epilepsy-rlated structural brain changes), biological [epilepsy-related changes in hypothalamic-pituitary axis (HPA), hormones, neurotransmitters and neuropeptides] mechanisms [27-29]as well as an adverse effect of AEDs are all contributed[24-26]. It seems to be a shared pathophysiological mechanisms caused by impairment of cellular metabolism associated with the process of epileptogenesis and neuronal plasticity and changes in HPA, neurotransmitters and pathways due to epilepsy itself or or its treatment. Increasing GABAergic inhibitory activity, glutamate blockage activity, alteration of serotoninergic, adrenergic and noradrenergic neurotrasmitters and pathways might contribute to behavioral changes associated with AEDs.

In this article, a review of the literature was performed through searching in MEDLINE for articles published between 1990 and 2011 with the following search terms: behavioral/emotional/psychiatric comorbidities, suicide and epilepsy, aggression and epilepsy and antiepileptic medications and behavior.

Data of epidemiological, longitudinal, prospective, double-blinded and clinical trial studies were considered. We also checked the reference lists of the retrieved studies for additional reports of relevant studies. Studies whose results were published in a language other than English were excluded. We discussed the prevalences and the characterization of peri-ictal (pre-ictal, ictal and post-ictal) and inter-ictal behavioral abnormalities associated with epilepsy and their impacts of patients' quality of life. We discussed factors or variables correlated with the associated behavioral comorbidities (psychosocial, demographic-, clinical-, epilepsy-related and treatment-related variables). We also discussed the mechanisms of behavioral abnormalities in relation to epilepsy itself and its medications.This is followed by the proposed guidelines for biopsychosocial approach to manage a patient as a whole and not only concentrate on seizure control.

B. Characterization and Prevalences of Behavioral Comorbidities with Epilepsy

1) Peri-Ictal (Pre-Ictal, Ictal and Post-Ictal) Behavioral Symptomatologies

Nearly one third of patients, particularly patients with secondarily generalized seizures, develop *pre-ictal* prodromal symptoms hours to days before seizures.Prodromal symptoms include: alterations of mood, depression, abnormal emotions, irritability, restlessness or motor hyperactivity, ideation and poor frustration tolerance. Such symptoms often relieved by the occurance of convulsions or persist for few days. It has been suggested that these prodromal symptoms may represent a biophyiological processes involved in intiation of abnormal emotions and seizures or a subtle or subclinical seizure activity [5]. *Ictal* behavioral symptoms occur in approximately 25% of auras (particularly prolonged auras), following a cluster of complex partial and secondary generalized seizures of temporal lobe epilepsy (TLE) or non-convulsive status epilepticus [30]. Ictal behavioral symptoms include: depression (which ranges from mild feelings of sadness to profound hopelessness, despair feelings of anhedonia, guilt and suicidal ideation) [5], fear, distres, nervousness, anger, irritability, panic attacks, phobias [6,31] forced thinking, obcession [12,13] and aggression [8]. Depressed mood and fear were reported as an aura in approximately 1% and 10–15%. Ictal behavioral symptoms tend to be of sudden onset, stereotyped, paroxysmal, of brief duration and unprovoked by environmental stimuli. They are sometimes associated with other characteristics of temporal discharges such as depersonalization and déja vu, as well as automatism which are manifested as altered consciousness, bizarre behaviour, mutism and amnesia [32]. *Post-ictal* behavioral symptoms usually occur after a volley of seizures, particularly with TLE and last hours to days. Post-ictal behavioral symptoms include depression with variable severity (even suicide), pure anxiety or anxiety with dysphoria or depression, psychosis and transient aggression [7,33,34]. Aggression is frequently observed in post-ictal confusional states or post-ictal psychoses. Aggression associated with epilepsy can be discriminated from a non-ictally related event by its directionality, for example: in ictal aggression, planned and focused aggression is not of ictal origin; however, ictal aggression might ensue if postictal delirium is forcibly contained [16,32]. Post-ictal psychosis (PIP) represents 25% of psychotic disorders seen in patients with epilepsy [33].PIPis characterized by: *a)* psychotic or other psychiatric symptoms occur after a seizure or more frequently after a series of seizures, with a delay [ranging between 12 hours up to 5-7 days of the seizure(s)] between the onset of psychiatric symptoms and the time of the lastseizure, *b)* an increase in the frequency of secondarily generalized tonic-colonicseizures preceding the onset of PIP, *c)* PIP is relatively of short duration, lasting from a few hours, days, or rarely weeks (up to 3-4 weeks), *d)* manifestations may be psychosis, depression, elation, or anxietyand clustering of symptoms into delusional and affective-like psychosis. PIP is characterized by well-systematized delusions and hallucinations in a setting of preserved orientation and alertness which distinguish it from post-ictal confusion, *e)* a prompt response to low-dose neuroleptic medications or benzodiazepines. It has been suggested that post-ictal psychiatric manifestations are a direct manifestation of epileptic discharges in the brain, but may be a consequence of the inhibitory mechanisms involved in the termination of seizures [7,32,33].

2) Inter-Ictal Behavioral Symptomatologies and Disorders

Inter-ictal behavioral symptomatologies are frequently mild, spontaneously reversible, do not need medical intervention and not included in any specific diagnostic category defined by the Diagnostic and Statistical Manual of Mental Disorders Fourth Edition, Text Revision (DSM IV TR) published by the American Psychiatric Association (2000). However, some patients with interactable epilepsy have enduring symptoms that fully meet the criteria of mood (as depression, mania, mixed and rapid cycling), anxiety (as panic attacks, phobias, generalized anxiety), personality (as epileptic characteropathi), schizophreniform psychosis, impulse controlling (irritability-aggression), somatoform (pain, conversion, somatization), associative(as dissociative amnesia, fugue) disorders, psychogenic non-epileptic seizures and mixed psychopathological symptoms. *Table (1)* shows the prevalence of different inter-ictal psychiatric comorbidities with epilepsy.However, it is obvious that there are big differences in rates for psychiatric disorders across studies reflecting the cultural differences or different risk factors across populations.

Depression is the most frequent psychiatric disorder in patients with epilepsy, with prevalence of 20-55% and sometimes up to 80% [35,36] compared to 1.5-19% in the general population [37]. Most studies reported higher risk among males with epilepsy than female. In contrast, data from general population show that the rates of major depression and dysthymia are higher in females than in males [20].

Depression in epilepsy may manifest as: *i)* Major depressive disorder and dysthymia meeting Diagnostic and Statistical Manual, 4th edition (DSM-IV); *ii)* Atypical depression or dysthymia with a fluctuating course and a pleomorphic presentation as depressive moods, prominent irritability, intermixed with euphoric mood, fear and symptoms of anxiety, anergia, pain and insomnia. In severe form, this disorder may become associated with intense depressive mood and with psychotic features (hallucinations, paranoia, delusions or bizarre behaviour) and even sudden suicide attempts may occur; and *iii)* A dysthymic-like disorder with intermittent symptoms that is milder than those of major depression [9, 38, 39].

Table 1. The prevalence of different inter-ictal psychiatric comorbidities with epilepsy

Psychiatric comorbidities	Epileptic population	General population
Depression disorder	17.4-80%	1.5-19%
Mania, hypomania and manic-depressive illness	3.03-8.25%	0.3-1.5%
Anxiety	19-66%	19.6%
Obsessive–compulsive disorder	14- 22%	2-13%
Attention-deficit-hyperactivity disorder	30-40%	15%
Personality traits and disorders	21.15%	5.9- 13.4%
Psychosis	6–10%	1-7%
Suicide	13-25%	1.4-6.9%,

Mania, hypomania and manic-depressive illness are rarely associated with epilepsy with prevalence of 3.03-8.25% [10,40] compared to 0.3-1.5% in general population [41]. A US survey demonstrated that biopolar symptoms to be present in ~12.2% of patients with epilepsy which is twice than than those with asthma and seven times as those of general population (~2%) [42]. The major symptoms of interictal dysphoric disorder has been defined by Blumer [43] as follow: 1) labile depressive symptoms: as anergia, depressed mood, insomnia and pain, 2) labile affective symptoms: as anxiety and fear, 3) specific symptoms as euphoric mood and paroxysmal irritability.

Anxiety is the second most common psychiatric disorders in adults with epilepsy after depression with prevalence ranges from 19 to 25% or up to 66% [11] which is higher than in the general population (~19.6%) [44]. Coexistance of inter-ictal anxiety and depression is not unusual (73%) in patients with epilepsy [32]. Anxiety disorders in epilepsy may manifest as generalized anxiety disorder, panic disorder, phobias, obsessive compulsive disorder, and posttraumatic stress disorder. Some people with epilepsy develop anticipatory anxiety of the attacks in public and may become agoraphobic [11].

Obsessive–compulsive symptoms (OCSs) and disorder (OCD) are not infrequent in patients with epilepsy with prevelance of 14-22%, particularily in TLE [13], compared to 2-13% in the general population [45]. OCD is characterized by recurrent intrusive and unpleasant thoughts often allied with compulsive actions. Studies suggested a causal relationship between epilepsy and the development of OCSs. Some authors considered them as part of an epileptic aura in TLE (e.g. a variant of epileptiform forced thinking) [46]. Also several authors suggested the existence of a specific temporal lobe behavioral syndrome including hyposexuality, religiosity, obsessional traits, compulsive writing or hypergraphia and marked philosophical interests [47, 48].

Attention-deficit-hyperactivity disorder (ADHD) occurs frequently in children and adults with severe epilepsy. At least 20% of children with epilepsy have clinical ADHD compared to 3% to 7% of the general pediatric population [49]. Clinical studies suggest that 30-40% of adults with epilepsy also have ADHD [14] compared to 15% in general population [50]. Symptoms of ADHD with epilepsy is diagnostically distinct from primary ADHD as inattention is more severe and frequent than impulsivity/hyperactivity and attention problems may predate the onset of epilepsy and is frequently associated with cognitive deficits [14].

Personality traits and disorders are frequent in patients with epilepsy. The prevalence of personality disorders in patient with epilepsy is about 21.15% [51] or even higher in patients with TLE and in patients who have undergone surgery [15] compared to 5.9- 13.4% in general population [52]. Dependent and avoidant personality disorders are by far the most common diagnoses, others include: antisocial, obsessive–compulsive, schizoid, schizotypal, dependent and dissociated personality. Earlier studies identified specific personality characteristics among patients with epilepsy, including: obsessional traits and marked philosophical interests. However, different types of epilepsy may be associated with different forms of abnormal thinking or behavior. Some studies reported that people with patients with frontal lobe epilepsy has characterstic personality profile compared to patients with TLE with more elevations on scales assessing emotional lability and relationship difficulties (i.e., mania, borderline features, antisocial, stress, and nonsupport) in associated with frontal lobe epilepsy [53].A chronic atypical psychosis with paranoid and affective features is more common in epileptic population (approximately 7% of epileptics) particularly with a definite temporal lobe focus. Some patients with intractable epilepsy develop high neuroticism, particularly when accompanied by lower extraversion, predisposed to poor adjustment to intractable epilepsy and reflected by impaired mood[54]. Geschwind [48] defined a collection of behavioral abnormalities that are associated with TLE which include: viscosity, circumstantiality, hypergraphia, and less frequently hyperreligiosity. In patients with juvenile myoclonic epilepsy (JME), some characterstic personality traits have been identified, which include: lack self-control, emotional instability with frequent and rapid mood changes and immaturity, lack of discipline, unsteadiness, indifference toward one's disease, sometimes appear to neglect of physical needs, poorly compliant with therapy, And sometimes become obstinate, bragging, impressionable, versatile and adaptable. The rapid comprehension and judgement, impressionability, open-mindedness, and awareness to the point of being easily distracted observed in some patients with JME, although give the impression that those patients are alert and intelligent, however, such characterstics are sometime problematic particularly with tasks that requir resoluteness, patience, and perseverance [55].

The prevalence of *psychosis* in the population of epilepsy ranges from 6–10%, and it is higher in patients with TLE and poorly controlled seizures [12] and patients who had multiple episodes of postictal psychosis before developing interictal psychosis [56] compared to 1-7% in general population [57]. Inter-ictal psychotic symptoms include: chronic non-episodic schizophrenia like psychosis, most commonly like paranoid schizophrenia with auditory and visual hallucinations and delusions (which are usually self-limiting and may last for few weeks), hyper-sexuality and aberrant philosophical or religious preoccupation. Inter-ictal psychosis may be associated with clouding of consciousness, confusion, disorientation, or delirium and delusions and hallucinations appear if consciousness is unimpaired. However, it has to be kept in mind that confusion may also be a symptom of very frequent absences or generalized inter-ictal epileptic discharges or toxicity from AEDs.In addition, persistent interictal psychoses of epilepsy and the schizophrenia-like psychoses of epilepsy have to be distinguished from traditional schizophrenia by the following [12]: *a)* lack of negative symptoms of schizophrenia, particularly flattening of affect and personality deterioration, *b)* better premorbid personality, *c)* paranoid delusions, *d)* delusions of reference, and *e)* more benign and variable course.

Aggressive behavior is among the frequent psychiatric comorbidity identified in patient with epilepsy, with prevalence varies between 4.8 - 50% (not taking into account the specific epileptic sub-syndromes) compared to aggression in general population with respection to specific socio-economic profile, public and family era and ethnic social vulnerabilities [8]. It may be seen as episodic aggression (is also defined as episodic dyscontrol) independent of observable ictal activity or in association with major psychiatric disorder or antisocial personality disorder [32].

Suicide and suicidality (suicidal thoughts and attempts) are frequent in the population of epilepsy with anestimated lifetime prevalence rate varies between 3.3 and 14.3% or even up to 32.5%. This rate has been reported to be 6 to 25 times higher in people with TLE [17,58-60] compared to 1.4-6.9% in the general population [61] and even higher for those who have had surgical treatment [62].It has been also found that suicide accounts for more than 10% of all deaths in people with epilepsy (compared with 1.4% in the general population) [63].Standardized mortality ratios were estimated for suicide in people with epilepsy and found to be between 3.3 and 13.9 [60]. In the meta-analysis study of Bell et al. [60], the authors estimated the risk suicide in people with epilepsy and the number of person-years at risk. The authors identified an overall standardized mortality ratios (SMRs) of 3.3 (95% CI 2.8-3.7) with significant increase with incident or newly diagnosed epilepsy in the community (SMR 2.1), populations with mixed prevalence and incidence cases (SMR 3.6), those with prevalent epilepsy (SMR 4.8), people in institutions (SMR 4.6), those seen in tertiary care clinics (SMR 2.28), with TLE (SMR 6.6), after temporal lobectomy (SMR 13.9), and following other forms of epilepsy surgery (SMR 6.4). The SMR was significantly low overall in two community-based studies of people with epilepsy and developmental disability.

Table 2. Epilepsy-related risks or correlates for developing inter-ictal psychiatric disorders

Psychosocial correlates	Low socio-economic status and poor cultural approach to epilepsy Poorer academic achievement and the lower the expectations of parents and teachers Unemployment Inability to drive, Low self-esteem, lessened well-being, social isolation and stigmatization Marital stresses and diminished sexual desire and responsiveness
Demographic, clinical- and epilepsy-related correlates Structural mechanisms Biological mechanisms	Type of epilepsy (temporal and frontal) Prolonged aura Frequency, severity andintractability of seizures Lateralization of foci Cause of seizure Recurrent epileptiform discharges, kindling and related neurobiological abnormalities Hypometabolism of specific brain areas Abnormal neuronal plasticity Cognitive deficits Dysfunction of some brain areas and pathways which include limbic system, temporal lobe, frontal lobe, orbitofrontal regions, anterior insula, anterior cingulate gyrus, amygdala, basal ganglia and periaqueductal grey matter Dysfunctions of the limbic system, frontal–limbic–subcortical circuits, frontal-striatal systems, limbic-brainstem connections or amygdale and its connections (e.g. amygdale-hypothalamic, amygdale-locus coeruleus) Cerebral GABA, catacholamines, dopaminergic, nonadrenergic, and serotonergic systems dysfunction
Other common pathogenic mechanisms	Historical predisposition to psychiatric disorders A genetic vulnerability or family history of psychiatric disorder Premorbid personality Endocrine and/or metabolic effects of seizures Sleep disturbance due to seizure Substance abuse

C.The Risks or Correlates for Developing Inter-ictal Psychiatric Disorders in Patients with Epilepsy

The risks for developing inter-ictal psychiatric manifestations in patients with epilepsy are multiple, both functional (psychogenic) and organic risks (epilepsy-related changes in the brain structure, neurotransmitters and pathways) are contributed.

In addition, some antiepileptic medications have behavioral risk profile. Thus, it is often difficult to singulate the etiology of the psychiatric symptomatologies. Table (2) summarizes the epilepsy-related risks or correlates for developing inter-ictal psychiatric disorders.

1) Psychosocial-Related Correlates

Psychosocial correlates are defined as the psychological response to epilepsy and its associated mental, physical and social challenges.

In general, behavioral disturbances seen in patients with epilepsy are more closely related to the overall function and well-being of the patient rather than seizure frequency and severity.

The poor adjustment to seizures, low socio-economic status, financial stress, poor cultural approach to epilepsy, poorer academic achievement, the lower the expectations of parents and teachers,unemployment (with rates up to 50% in developed countries if seizures are not fully controlled and up to 100% in developing countries), inability to drive, marital stresses, diminished sexual desire and responsiveness, all result in a negative effect on effort and attitude about his or her abilities, low self-esteem, lessened well-being, social isolation, stigmatization, depression and other psychiatric abnormalities and a lower quality of life [18,19].

On the other hand, the presence of negative, depressed or dysphoric mood in combination with negative life events may increase the likelihood of seizures. The association between epilepsy and depression is also related to poor performance on measures of cognition and behavior and increase the risk of suicide [64]. In fact, it has been found that the earlier onset (below the age of 18) and longer duration of epilepsy, the better quality of life in adult patients.

This reflects the more effective copying mechanisms and the adjustment to the social and psychological consequences of the disease. While the late onset seizures may be more disruptive to patients' life, for example: due to loss of the ability to drive and unemployment [18]. Anxiety may result as responses to the unpredictability of seizures and fear of the unknown or fear of death.

This results in restrictions on normal living and activities, stigmatization and social rejection, misinformation about the disorder and low self-esteem [9]. On the other hand, any people find that periods of anxiety and stress increase the frequency of seizures [65].

Personality disorders in patients with epilepsy could be an adaptation or reaction to psychosocial variables such fears of embarrassment, stigmatization, reluctance to engage in social interaction and over-dependency caused by parental overprotection, low self-esteem, poor social adaptation, social isolation, fewer friends, failure to establish good sexual relationships, a lower likelihood of marriage, marital distress and depression. This results in hypochondria and misbehaviors as well as erroneous self-perception, self-aversion and anti-social behavior.

The unpredictability of the epileptic attack and the fear of unknown cause it easy to deny the illness and poor compliance to treatment [15]. Aggression may result as a consequence of depression, anxiety or in the context of an antisocial personality disorder [32].

Suicidality (thoughts and attempts) is associated with certain psychiatric comorbidity as decreased adaptive abilities, depression, increased emotional problems and a combination of pronounced epileptoid type personality changes [17].

2) Demographic-, Clinical- and Epilepsy-related Correlates

a) Characterization of the Inter-ictal Behavioral/emotional Symptomatologies and Disorders and the Mechanisms of its Cauation in Relation to Epilepsy itself

In general, type, frequency and severity of seizures, lateralization of foci, cause of seizure, long-term effect of repeated seizures are risk factors for psychiatric disorders in patients with epilepsy.

The risk of *depression* was found to be highest in individuals with TLE, frequent seizures or refractory epilepsy [66,67]. The majority of the studies implicate the left sided foci (2-3 folds higher than right sided foci) as a potential risk factor for depression, particularly left sided TLE in association with frontal lobe hypofunction [67]. Some studies implicate the right hemisphere as a risk of depression in epileptic patients and suggested that this might be attributed to the extensive limbic connections than the left hemisphere. Others found no effect of lateralization at all [68]. The risk of *anxiety* is higher in focal than in generalized epilepsies, TLE, frontal lobe epilepsy, severe epilepsy, high seizure frequency, chronic refractory seizure disorders and first onset seizure late in life [68]. *OCD* is seen most often in TLE, frontal lobe seizures originating in the anterior cingulate gyrus or near the corpus callosum [69]. Cognitive deficits, particularily memory defect, and organizational deficulties, due to frontal lobe dysfunctions, are observed in patients with TLE, and/or OCD[13]. Some studies reported a link between OCD and seizures originating from the left cerebral hemisphere [70]. The risk of *personality traits and disorders* are highin TLE, severe epilepsy, high seizure frequency, chronic refractory seizure disorders and left sided foci, longer duration of illness, premorbid personality and presence of other psychiatric disorders as mood or emotional changes [51,53]. *Psychotic disorders* in patients with epilepsy have been found to be related to several epilepsy-related variables which include: *1)* type of seizure (as TLE and fronal lobe epilepsies) [51], lateralization of foci (as left sided foci) and presence of more auras, cause of seizure as mesial temporal lobe, earlier onset of epilepsy and longer duration of illness, cognitive deficits and poor intellectural functions and genetic factor and family history of psychosis [71-74]. *ADHD* in epilepsy is related to several factors which include: frontal lobe dysfunction, long-term effects of repeated seizures and and genetic factors [75,76]. The risk of *aggressive behavior* in epilepsy has been found to be frequently related to left TLE, intractable epilepsy, a low intelligence quotient in particular verbal intelligence, early onset of seizures, a dominant-hemisphere electroencephalographic (EEG) focus and antisocial personality disorders [32]. The risk of *suicide behavior* in epilepsy is related to several variables which include: male sex [77], early age of onset of seizures [78],TLE, high frequency of primary generalized seizures, polymorphic seizures combination [79] and a more severe epilepsy [80], lateralization of the epileptic focus [78], recent control of seizures, absence of seizures for a long time, especially after being very frequent [80], cognitive deterioration and hypofrontality [81] and psychiatric comorbidity [59,60,82]. Retrospective studies indicate that the absolute majority (81–100%) of suicides occurs in subjects with a psychiatric illness, depression being the most common diagnosis with a risk reaching about 15%-18.9%, and in some studies it may be as high as 50 times that of the general population. Other psychiatric comorbidities include anxiety, mixed anxiety and mood or affective disorder and combination of pronounced epileptoid type personality changes [64]. Others risks include past history of mood and anxiety disorders, family history of psychiatric disorders, particularly when associated with suicidal behavior, past suicidal attempts and the continual availability of agents (as AEDs) [59,80].

b) Mechanisms of Inter-ictal Behavioral/emotional Symptomatologies and Disorders in Relation to Epilepsy-related Correlates

There seems to be a bidirectional relationship between epilepsy and psychiatric disorders indicating that both disorders share the same neuroanatomic structures, common pathogenic mechanisms and common neurotransmitters. Recurrent epileptiform discharges, kindling, and related neurobiological abnormalities will result in prolonged aura, hypometabolism of other brain areas, abnormal neuronal plasticity, epilepsy intractability cognitive deficits and behavioral phenomena [21,23,26,68,83].

i) Structural Mechansims

Behavioral impairment may be related to the pathological nature of the underlying cerebral dysfunctions and its effects on brain structure and function. In general, the epilepsy process e.g. epileptogenesis and the abnormal recurrent synaptic bombardment of distant projection areas, caused by repeated focal or generalized ictal and inter-ictal epileptiform discharges may induce plastic changes (sensory-limbic hyper-connection) through kindling mechanisms and impair the naturally occurring homeostatic which maintain the inter-ictal state with adverse consequences on the normal neuronal and psychological functions [21,83,84].

There is evidence of a causal relationship between behavioral disorders, and pathological dysfunction in a variety of brain areas. The following brain areas are incriminated in generating both epileptic discharges and behavioral symptoms, they include: limbic system, temporal lobe, frontal lobe, orbitofrontal regions, anterior insula, anterior cingulate gyrus, amygdala, basal ganglia and periaqueductal grey matter [22,23,75,85]. Dysfunctions of the limbic system, frontal–limbic–subcortical circuits, frontal-striatal systems, limbic-brainstem connections or amygdale and its connections (e.g. amygdale-hypothalamic, amygdale-locus coeruleus) are the most important causes of behavioral disorders in patients with epilepsy [21,86,87]. Epileptogenic lesions which are able to disrupt limbic connections as inHS and TLE are at increased risk for development of cognitive and behavioral disorders compared to those with extra-temporal or primary generalized epilepsies. It has been suggested that the Geschwind syndrome may be associated with an active focus in the temporal lobe producing a progressive change in the limbic structures and creating new pathways between these structures and the neocortex [47].

For *depression*, there is growing evidence in the literature that depression might be linked to small hippocampal volumes (i.e., HS itself appeared to be the main factor associated with the occurrence of depression) [66,88,89]. This may explain why some studies found that the frequancy of seizures didn't correlate with severity of depression, and seizure-free state couldn't protect the epileptic patients from developing a depression and consequently, suicidality. It has also been detected that in patients with epilepsy, temporal lobe dysfunction may result in hypo-metabolism of extratemporal regions as the frontal lobe and frontal lobe dysfunction increases the vulnerability to depression [89]. The hypo-perfusion (hypo-metabolism) observed in the limbic frontal regions in patients with TLE may be related to inter-ictal inhibitory activity, post-ictal depletion of substrates (decreased levels of neurotransmitters) or functional differentiation.In support [89,90]: *1)* a bilateral reduction in inferior frontal lobe glucose metabolism on positron emission tomography (PET) scans was observed in patients with depression and TLE, *2)* reduced activity measured with single photon emission computed tomography (SPECT) in bilateral frontal and right temporal regions was associated with higher scores on the Beck Depression Index in patients with left TLE [91]. Abnormalities of metabolism in the amygdala and anterior cingulate gyrus have also been reported to be associated with depression and TLE [90]. In addition, the presence of connections between limbic structures and brainstem nuclei with opioid projections to the forebrain and the observation that endogenous opioid peptides (endogenous euphorogens) are elevated during seizures and mu-opiate-receptor binding is increased in TLE, might suggest that patients suffering from frequent limbic seizures might develop dependence to high levels of circulating opioids, and affective symptoms reflect a form of withdrawal when seizures do not regularly recur and thus, depression and other abnormalities observed in patients with epilepsy [21].

For *anxiety*, the amygdala seems to be a particularly important structure for the production of anxiety symptoms and epileptic discharges in TLE [92,93]. In support: *1)* More than 50% of patients with magnetic resonance emaging (MRI)-confirmed amygdala atrophy on the same side as the seizure focus, have some form of ictal fear [85], *2)* Patients with TLE and ictal anxiety symptoms have been found to have a reduced amygdala volume [68], *3)* The amygdala may provide the affective tone to perceptions and experiences. The projections of the central nucleus of the amygdala to the locus coeruleus and hypothalamus have been found to be responsible for the arousal and autonomic responses associated with fear and anxiety which together with the function of amygdala in emotion recognition and fear conditioning, imply a key role of the amygdala in the integration of behavioral and neuroendocrine components of the stress response [92], *4)* Human lesions and functional and structural neuroimaging studies demonstrate the role of the amygdala in verbal and non-verbal recognition of emotions as well as fear-induced anxiety, provoked anxiety and panic disorders. Other structures correlated with anxiety are the orbitofrontal cortex, anterior insula and anterior cingulate gyrus [92,93].

OCD in patients with epilepsy may be due to structural damage to specific frontal–limbic–subcortical circuits [13]. There is evidence of a causal relationship between obsessive compulsive symptoms, and pathological dysfunction in a variety of brain areas, for example, limbic system, basal ganglia, and orbitofrontal regions, generating both epileptic discharges and obsessive compulsive symptoms. Paroxysmal epileptic discharges from the frontal and limbic brain regions may make patients particularly susceptible to obsessive compulsive behavior, as seizures localized to one area of the brain stimulate another area (such as the limbic region) and lead to the emergence of obsessive-compulsive behaviour. Also the amygdala seems to be crucial to affective and motivational elements of OCD.The amygdala has dense connections with the striatum that are presumed to support an efficient system for driving automated behavior in response to danger, while reciprocal connections with the extended amygdala, including the ventral striatum and the bed nucleus of the stria terminalis, may help to mediate the anxiolytic by-products of repetitive behaviors [93].

The most important brain structures implicated in the mediation of *aggressive behaviour* being the amygdala and associated limbic structures, the frontal lobes, periaqueductal grey and the hypothalamus. Within this network of critical structures, the amygdala is thought to play a crucial role in the mediation of fear induced aggression [94].

ADHD in patients with epilepsy may be due to frontal lobe dysfunction and fronto-striatal system. In support: *1)* frontal lobe epilepsy shares behavioral features with ADHD, presenting with impulsivity, disinhibition, and excitement/irritability [75,76], *2)* Abnormally increased volume of frontal lobe gray matter, as measured by voxel-based morphometry, has been found in patients with ADHD. Regions of increased gray matter volume are located in sensorimotor, supplementary motor and prefrontal regions, areas congruent with the core neuropsychological abnormalities in motor/psychomotor processing and attention/execution function [95], *3)* Positron and single-photon emission tomography scan have also indicated hypofunction and low metabolic activity in the brain at prefrontal and caudate nucleus areas (frontal-striatal systems) [95,96]. These abnormalities may be associated with difficulties in planning, judgment, and time perception. In addition, in patients with ADHD, abnormally reused brainstem volume has been identified, given the role of the reticular activating system and several neurotransmitters originating in and around the brainstem in causation of ADHD [97].

ii) Biological Mechanisms

The correlation of behavioral disturbances and epilepsy may be explained by the role of GABA theory.GABA is the most important inhibitory transmitter in the CNS. Decreased activity of GABA neurotransmitter or abnormal functioning of GABA receptors have been shown to facilitate the kindling process of seizure foci, to exacerbate seizure severity, and to intensify seizure predisposition in some animal models of epilepsy, depression, anxiety and to less extent psychosis symptomatologies. A hyperactive hypothalamic-pituitary-adrenal (HPA) axis, cerebral GABA, catacholamines, dopaminergic, nonadrenergic, and serotonergic systems dysfunction play pivotals role in the expression of depression, anxiety; psychosis, ADHD and suicide [29,98,99]. In some patients, with epilepsy and depression, decreased serotonergic and noradrenergic functions or alteration of dopaminergic activity were identified as pivotal pathogenic mechanisms [98]. Preclinical and clinical studies suggest that 5-hydroxytryptamine 1A (5-HT1A) receptors play a role in the pathophysiology of both TLE, depressive and anxiety disorder [100].

In patients with epilepsy and psychosis, it has also been suggested that neurophysiological modifications such as seizure-suppressive inhibitory mechanisms that develop gradually in chronic epilepsy may alter dopaminergic activity and contribute to the risk for the development of psychosis in patients with epilepsy. In addition, ionic currents, opiates, adenosine, glutamate and nitric oxide might also play a role in psychosis related to epilepsy. It has also been hypothesized that epilepsy-related psychoses may partially result from excessive hippocampal dynorphin release and kappa opioid receptor over stimulation which aims to seizure control [101]. Epilepsy and ADHDmay share a common underlying deficit in the central norepinephrine and dopaminergic systems, but the exact mechanism remains elusive [102]. Other proposed mechanisms include: underlying neurodevelopmental disorder and common genetic defects. Analysis of the literature has shown that serotonin metabolism disturbances are involved in the pathogenesis of suicidal behaviour irrespective of primary diagnosis. Serotonin disturbances also seem to be a common link between depression, suicidality and even epilepsy itself [103,104]

Table 3. Summary of the currently available antiepileptic drugs (AEDs) and their mechanisms of action

AEDs	Mechanism(s) of action
PB	PB directly binds to $GABA_A$/benzodiazepine receptor complexes (GBRs). PB augments the inhibitory effect of GABA by prolonging the chloride-channel opening at the GABA-A receptors.
BZ	Directly binds to GABA/Cl- channel complex, potent GABA agonists.
PHT	PHT blocks voltage dependent neuronal sodium channels. Thereby limiting rapid repetitive neuronal firing and controls the excitatory synaptic transmission.
CBZ	CBZ blocks voltage dependent neuronal sodium channels. Thereby limiting rapid repetitive neuronal firing and controls the excitatory synaptic transmission.
VPA	VPA Indirectly modulates GABA neurotransmissions. VPA enhances $GABA_A$ receptor-mediated hyperpolarizing responses. VPA reduces low threshold (T-type) calcium currents and blocks voltage-dependent sodium channels.
OXC	OXC is the prodrug for its active metabolite, 10,11-dihydro-10-hydroxycarbazepine, which blocks voltage-dependent sodium channels, and modulates calcium and potassium currents.
ETX	ETX causes blockage of low threshold (T-type) calcium channels
VGB	VGB is an analogue of GABA. VGB elevates brain GABA several-fold by irreversibly inhibiting the GABA-metabolizing enzyme, GABA-transaminase.
GBP	The exact antiepileptic mechanism of action of GBP is not known. GBP indirectly modulates of GABA neurotransmission. GBP enhances the levels of GABA in the brain and decreases brain glutamate concentration. Its actions include modulation of GABA synthesizing enzyme, glutamic acid decarboxylase (GAD) and glutamate synthesizing enzyme, branched-chain amino acid transaminase. GBP demonstrates effects on voltage-gated ion channels (sodium and calcium), presynaptic mechanisms can enhance GABAergic inhibition, and ligand-gated ion channels (GABA receptors and glutamate receptors). GBP binds to the $\alpha 2\delta$ subunit of neuronal voltage-gated calcium channels, inhibiting calcium flow.
TGB	TGB induces its effect by increasing synaptic GABA availability via selective inhibition of the GAT-1 GABA transporter. It inhibits neuronal and glial reuptake of GABA, which increases the availability of GABA to inhibit postsynaptic neurons.
TPM	TPM enhances GABAergic neurotransmission. TPM has sodium channel blockage activity. It has inhibitory effect on carbonic anhydrase isoenzymes II and IV, causing increased Mg^{++}-dependent tonic inhibition of NMDA receptors. It has negative modulatory effect on the AMPA/KA subtype of glutamate receptors
LTG	The precise mechanism by which LTG exerts its therapeutic effect is unknown. LTG inhibits voltage-sensitive sodium channels, thereby stabilizing neuronal membranes and consequently modulating presynaptic transmitter release of excitatory amino acids.
LEV	Its exact mechanism of action is unknown. LEV binds to synaptic vesicle protein and has actions on neuronal GABA and glycine-gated currents, as well as voltage-dependent potassium currents.

AEDs	Mechanism(s) of action
ZNS	The exact mechanism of action is not known for ZNS. ZNS may be a carbonic anhydrase inhibitor. Its mechanism of action might be through blocking repetitive firing of voltage-gated sodium channels and reduction of T-type calcium channel currents, or by binding allosterically to GABA receptors like the BZ and muscimol, or increasing the levels of the glutamate transport protein in the brain while decreasing the amount of GABA transport protein.
FBM	FBM potentiates GABA-mediated inhibition and blocks voltage-dependent sodium channels as well as the ionic channels at the NMDA receptors.

Phenobarbital (PB), vigabatrin (VGB), and topiramate (TPM), zonisamide (ZNC), tiagabin (TGB), levitracetam (LEV) and felbamate (FBM), Phenytoin (PHT), carbamazepine (CBZ), oxcarbazepine (OXC), gabapentin (GBP), valproate (VPA) and lamotrigine (LTG), Ethosuximide (ETX)

It has been found that a history of attempted suicide is five times more common in newly diagnosed epilepsy patients [64], and a history of depression is 1.7–7 times more common in newly diagnosed epilepsy patients [64]. Patients with major depression are six-fold more likely to have an unprovoked seizure than the general population [105]. Because there is a closer link between breathing and 5-HT neuron dysfunction, it has been suggested that there are reasons to believe that a defect in 5-HT neurons could lead to sudden unexpected death with epilepsy (SUDEP). A reduction in firing activity of 5-HT neurons during and after a seizure could lead to ictal and/or postictal hypoventilation and SUDEP, particularly in genetically susceptible individuals [104].

iii) Other Common Pathogenic Mechanisms between Behavioral/Emotional Disturbances and Epilepsy

Historical predisposition to psychiatric disorders, a genetic vulnerability or family history of psychiatric disorder, premorbid personality, cognitive impairment, substance abuse [106], endocrine and/or metabolic effects of seizures [107] and sleep disturbance due to seizurs.

3) Treatment-Related Correlates

a) Characterization of Inter-ictal Behavioral/Emotional Symptomatologies and Disorders and Mechanisms of its Cauation in Relation to Antiepileptic Medications

Some AEDs have demonstrated mood improvement (positive psychotropic effect) and may have therapeutic potential for epilepsy population. However, other AEDs may result in behavioural disorders (negative psychotropic effect) in patients with epilepsy [24-26]. In general,the positive or negative psychotropic effects of AEDs are probably related both to direct and indirect mechanisms.AEDs are directly able to improve behavior because of their *antiseizure effect* through altering ion channels and neurotransmitter system functions (i.e. GABA enhancement or glutamate antagonism) [108], and modulation the electrochemical systems or indirectly through *a release phenomenon* in which successful seizure control with AED is associated with a positive impact on alertness and cognition. On the other hand, the iatrogenic behavioral disturbances (negative psychotropic effect) associated with AEDs may result from *the main properties of the drug* (alteration of ion channels and neurotransmitter system functions and modulation the electrochemical systems) [24-26,108], or indirectly from the effect of the drug on the epilepsy itself or epilepsy-related phenomena, i.e. *forced normalization phenomenon* in which successful seizure control with AED is associated with negative impact on behavior (i.e., worsening of behavior with improvement in seizure control). *Alternative psychosis* is also a term used to illustrate the inverse relationship between seizure control and the occurrence of psychotic symptoms. Alternative psychosis may occur as an iatrogenic effect of the AEDs [109]. The most frequent manifestation of alternative psychosis is a paranoid psychosis without clouding of consciousness and with a richness of affective symptoms [110].

Negative psychotropic effects associated with AEDs are complex and can vary dramatically between patients. However, it is currently not possible to predict which patient with epilepsy will tolerate an AED or develop positive or negative psychotropic effects. Behavioral effects of AEDs are commonly associated with rapid dose titration, slow drug metabolism, electrolyte and other metabolic derangements (as folate deficiency) [111,112], polypharmacy and drug-drug interactions, drug toxicity and drug withdrawal [24].

Some AEDs drugs have a great risk for develping *depression*, which included: phenobarbital (PB) [113], vigabatrin (VGB) [114], tiagabin (TGB) [115], levitracetam (LEV) [116], felbamate (FBM) [117], zonisamide (ZNC) [118]and topiramate (TPM) [119].In some studies, PB, VGB and TPM show greater associations with the occurrence of depressive symptoms than other AEDs, presenting in up to 10% of all patients, but even more so in susceptible patients. Data on zonisamide (ZNC) [118] are scarce but it seems that mood disorders may occur in approximately 7% (intermediate risk) of patients who are receiving high dosages of this drug. TGB, LEV and FBM present a low risk, with prevalence of depression of about 4% or lower. PHT [120], carbamazepine (CBZ) [121], oxcarbazepine (OXC) [122,123], gabapentin (GBP) [124], valproate (VPA) [125,126] and lamotrigine (LTG) [127] are all associated with very low risks for depression (<1%).

Folate deficiency is another issue that might be of relevance regarding AEDs and depression. Patients on polytherapy are reported to have low serum, red cell or cerebrospinal fluid folate levels and this deficit seems to be even greater in patients with epilepsy and psychopathology. It is known that folic acid plays acrucial role in several important CNS transmethylation reactions and is linked to monoamine metabolism [111,112]. In this regard; it is worth noting that AEDs with a positive impact on mood and behavior, such as CBZ or LTG, have minimal effects on folate levels. On the contrary, it is established that PB or PHT treatment can depress serum, red blood cell, or CSF folate levels in a high proportion of patients and thus negative impact on mood [26]. Depressive disorder may occur following the discontinuation of AEDs with positive psychotropic properties, such as CBZ, OXC, VPA, or LTG. Also abrupt discontinuation of anticonvulsants can also cause acute psychosis. Also non-pharmacological treatments as surgery (particularly the first 6 months after epilepsy surgery) and vagus nerve stimulation have been suggested to have a role in the increased risk of psychiatric abnormalities and even suicide in epileptic patients with 5 times higher than patients in pharmacological therapy [62,128-130].The concept of forced normalization (or alternative psychosis), in which good control of seizures (regardless of control of EEG changes) results in appearance of behavioral abnormalities or psychosis has been suggested by many as a cause of mood adverse effects and even suicidal risk due to AEDs, epilepsy surgery and vagus nerve stimulation, although the exact mechanisms are not fully understood.AEDs may also contribute to the development of *anxiety*, either as a side effect or because of withdrawal [24]. The common AEDs implicated are the GABAergic drugs, such as PB, benzodiazepines (BZ), VPA, GBP and VGB.TPM, PHT, VPA, LTG, FBM, ZNC and VGB are common AEDs associated with *psychosis* [26]. AEDs play a role in increased risk of *suicide* in epileptic patients [131]. In the study of Kalinin and Polyanskiy [132], in search for risk factors of suicide behavior in epileptic patients, 105 patients were examined, including those with (n=70) and without (n=35) suicide behavior. The authors found that high frequency of primary generalized seizures and polymorphic seizures combination and typical anticonvulsants daily dosage, including PB, correlated with suicidal behavior, on the contrary, high frequency of complex partial seizures and high dosage of VPA derivatives and CBZ were found to benegatively correlated with a risk of suicidal behavior in epileptic patients. VPA derivatives, CBZ, LTG are superior in epilepsy treatment in prevention of suicidal behavior compared to PB and novel AEDs. The relationship between AEDs and suicidality is a matter of concern throughout the last decade. In January 2008, the FDA [133] issued an alert regarding the association between suicidality and AEDs, which was based on results of a meta-analysis that included data from 199 randomized clinical trials of 11 AEDs: carbamazepine (CBZ), felbamate (FBM), gabapentin (GBP), lamotrigine (LTG), levetracitam (LEV), oxcarbazepine (OXC), pregabalin (PGB), tiagabine (TGB), topiramate (TPM), valproate (VPA), and zonisamide (ZNC). The meta-analysis encompassed 43,892 patients treated for epilepsy, psychiatric disorders, and other disorders, predominantly pain. The FDA concluded that there was a statistically significant 1.80-fold increased risk of suicidality with exposure to AEDs. Suicidality occurred in 4.3 per 1,000 patients treated with AEDs in the active arm, compared with 2.2 per 1,000 patients in the comparison arm. The FDA has decided to insert suicide warnings in the package inserts of all AEDs.In contrast to FDA results, very recently, Machado et al. [134] recruited 130 patients with epilepsy who were followed up for the previous 5 years, the authors identified suicide risk with PB, primidone (PRM), phenytoin (PHT) and LTG but the increased of risk diminished or disappeared when psychiatric comorbidity and other well established risk factors for suicidality were analyzed. The authors also found significant proportion of patients with depressive episodes associated with TPM, PHT and LTG. The authors concluded that AEDs do not have an impact on suicidality. Thus, the physicians need to identify patients with increased risks of suicidality and the results of FDA meta-analysis must be considered with great caution, and more research is necessary. However, it has to be kept in mind that some people with epilepsy are more likely to develop psychiatric adverse effects with any AEDs, and these people should be followed closely whenever a new AED is introduced.

b) AEDs Are Divided Based on their Predominant Negative Psychotropic Profiles and Mode of Action as Follow (Tables 3 and 4)

i) Sedating (GABA-ergic) Drugs

Sedating (GABA-ergic drugs) include: PB, primidone, VPA, GBP, TGB and VGB and PGB. These drugs usually potentiate gamma-amino butyric acid (GABA) inhibitory neurotransmission. These pharmacological properties are either mediated through the interaction of drugs with the GABA receptor, through agonism at the GABA binding site, or through an increase in endogenous GABA [135]. TPM is considered an AED with mixed profile. However, GABAergic properties are likely to dominate its action [108]. Increase GABA-ergic activity cause fatigue, cognitive slowing, depression and other behavioral abnormalities and weight gain [26] (Table 4). For example: PBcan impair cognition, attention and motivation and depress mental and physical energy as well as mood. PB impair sexual function and desire andmost likely causes depression and suicidal ideation in patients with a family history of affective disorder [132]. Some studies denote PB to have the greatest behavioral toxic potential with dose related impairment in attention and reaction time, performance intelligence quotient (IQ) and short-term memory, as well as inducing a hyperkinetic syndrome in children [113]. Gradual conversion to a non-barbiturate AED in epileptic patients with depressed, irritable or aggressive manifestations may avoid the need for prescribing a psychotropic medication. VPA causes sedation and infrequently may cause cognitive impairment, irritability, depression, hyperactivity and aggressive behavior [125], GBP can cause irritability and agitation and minimal detrimental cognitive and behavioural side effects in patients with epilepsy [124]. TGB therapy may cause difficulties with concentration, language problems, depression, and additional psychiatric symptoms such as emotional lability, hallucinations and paranoia [115].

Table 4. The mechanisms of negative psychotropic effects of antiepileptic medications

Positive psychotropic effects	
Direct mechanisms	Anti-seizure effect through altering ion channels and neurotransmitter system functions (i.e. GABA enhancement or glutamate antagonism) and modulation the electrochemical systems.
Indirect mechanisms	A release phenomenon: successful seizure control with AED is associated with a positive impact on alertness and cognition.
Negative psychotropic effects	
Direct mechanisms	The main properties of the drug through alteration of ion channels and neurotransmitter system functions and modulation the electrochemical systems).
Indirect mechanisms	Epilepsy-related phenomena as: *Forced normalization phenomenon* in which successful seizure control with AED is associated with negative impact on behavior (i.e., worsening of behavior with improvement in seizure control). *Alternative psychosis* in which the inverse relationship between seizure control and the occurrence of psychotic symptoms
Others	Rapid dose titration Slow drug metabolism Polypharmacy Drug-drug interactions Drug toxicity Drug withdrawal Electrolyte disturbance metabolic derangements as folate deficiency

VGB use was found to be associated with increased occurrence of depression and psychosis. Agitation, irritability and disturbed behavior have also been reported with VGB. Hyperkinesia and agitation commonly occur in pediatric populations on VGB [114].

Depression is one of the chief treatment-emergent adverse events during TPM therapy. High rate of psychosis was also reported with TPM [119]. Related risk factors are a past psychiatric history, rapid titration schedule and severe forms of epilepsy.

ii) Activating (Anti-glutamatergic) Drugs

Anti-glutamatergic drugs include: FBM and LTG. These drugs usually attenuate glutamate excitatory neurotransmission (Table 4). Anti-glutamatergic drugs may cause anxiety, insomnia, and agitation. LTG may result insomnia, irritability, hyperactivity, and stereotypic or aggressive behavior. FBM has stimulant properties, which can cause anxiety, irritability, or insomnia [24,26,117, 136].

iii) Antiepileptic Drugs which Act on Serotonin, Catecholamines or other Unknown Neurotransmitters

There are at least five AEDs (CBZ, OXC, VPA, LTG and ZNS) which also exert effect upon level of serotonin receptors [24]. CBZ may cause irritability, impaired attention and behavioral problems in patients with existing behavioral difficulties. Its active metabolite carbamazepine-epoxide is partly responsible for the mild cognitive and psychomotor effects attributed to CBZ. Agitation and irritability are recognized in some patients with ZNS. Mild degrees of confusion, nervousness, abnormal thinking and fatigue have been reported with ZNS therapy. High rates of psychosis and depression have been noted between ZNC and TPM, indicating their shared action as carbonic anhydrase-inhibiting drugs [137].

iv) Antiepileptic Drugs with Unknown Mechanism for its Psychotropic Effects

PHT has cognitive and behavioral profiles similar to that of CBZ. However, PHT is implicated in dose-related decline in concentration, memory, visuomotor functions and mental speed, as well as generating anxiety, aggression, fatigue, and depression [137]. LEV is chemically related to the putative nootropic drug piracetam [138]. It has been reported that approximately 5 to 10 of adults taking LEV may exhibit irritability, hostility, nervusness, emotional lability, anxiety, depression, and other behavioral and cognitive disorders [116,123].

PHT and LEV have no serotonergic properties, may cause anxiety, impair mood and cognitive functions and cosequantly increased risk of suicide (suicidogenic). Ethosuximide (ETX) is used to treat absence seizures. It may cause confusion, sleep disturbances as insomnia, aggressive behavior, depression and rarely psychosis [139]. Forced normalization with ethosuximide may cause behavioral abnormalities [140].

D. The Biopsychosocial Approach to Manage Patients with Epilepsy and Behavioral Abnormalities

Behavioral/emotional symptoms in epilepsy seem to be often underestimated and unrecognized. There are two main factors that contribute to the under-recognition and inadequate treatment of behavioral/emotional changes for patients with epilepsy, which include: a) considering behavioral changes a part or result from the primary illness or its treatment, an increased difficulty in diagnosis because some psychiatric disorders (e.g. depression) in epilepsy appear different or have features that are attributed to epilepsy itself. Also at some occasions, differentiating between spontaneous fear and reactive fear (ie, reaction to the knowledge that a seizure may occur) is difficult. Fear and anxiety are often associated with simple partial seizures.

Panic disorder can produce paroxysmal symptoms, which can be confused with epileptic events and may go unrecognized in patients with epilepsy. Anxiety also may be related to non-epileptic attack disorder. In fact, the lack of well conducted studies demonstrating the effect of cognitive, behavioral or pharmacological therapies directed at psychiatric symptoms and disorders due to the lack of sufficient research information and controversial reports from different studies, it is currently not possible to predict which patient with epilepsy will tolerate an AED or develop positive or negative psychotropic effects [141].

For example, Goldstein et al. [142] found that patients with epilepsy with high seizure frequency had lower anxiety scores than those with lower seizure frequency, and b) an apparent lack of appreciation of the common occurrence and impact of psychiatric comorbidities and the failure to screen or even consider some psychiatric symptoms (e.g. depression) as an important issue for clinical care.

Thus, early recognition and treatment of inter-ictal disturbed behaviour might help patients and carers to cope more effectively with everyday life activities [16] as well as reducing seizure frequency. Several studies confirmed the bidirectional relationship between behavioral disorders and epilepsy, meaning that patients with epilepsy have an increased prevalence of behavioral symptomatologies and psychiatric disorders, while the latter increases seizure risk.

In the treatment of epilepsy related behavioral abnormalities, there are special considerations in pharmacologic intervention for patients; which include: 1) one must consider whether the psychiatric manifestations can be ascribed to seizures themselves, for example, treatment of psychiatric manifestations attributable to the prodromal and peri-ictal periods should be directed toward maximizing intervention with AEDs, 2) after determining that psychiatric manifestations are not directly related to a seizure, other possible risk factors should be evaluated before a psychotropic drug is prescribed. Example of these factors: psychosocial problems, side effects of AEDs, polypharmacy, folic acid deficiency associated with the use of AEDs and the phenomenon of "forced normalization" or "Alternative psychosis".

Some authors consider that alternative psychotic episodes should be treated by reducing or discontinuing AEDs until seizure recurrence causes a remission of psychotic symptoms. 3) After a thorough assessment of these factors, if a salient psychiatric symptom persists or the AED cannot be changed, both behavioral and pharmacologic intervention as antidepressant, anxiolytic or psychotropic drug should be started. However, some antidepressants, anxiolytics or antipsychotic drugs may manifest convulsant effects from decreasing the seizure threshold and thus cautious has to be paid to the epileptogenic potential, adverse effects, and drug interactions.

Treatment Strategies for Patients with Comorbid Epilepsy and Behavioral Abnormalities Are as Follow (Table 5)

1. Treatment of Peri-ictal Behavioral Symptomatology

Pre-ictal and ictal depression does not usually require treatment. Improvement in seizure frequency is expected to reduce its occurrence. Ictal abnormalities are treated in the same way as non-psychiatric epileptic events. Postictal events are treated by improving seizure control. Post-ictal depression may require small doses of antidepressants.So et al. [30] believe that PIP remits spontaneously even without treatment.Patients with PIP should not start daily doses of antipsychotic drugs and often the psychotic episode could be aborted or shortened in duration with a timely administration of low-dose neuroleptic drug such as risperidone, haloperidolor benzodiazepines.

2. Treatment of Inter-ictal Behavioral Symptomatology

a) Optimizing Seizure Control

Priority should be given to optimizing seizure control [143].

b) Psychotherapy, Counseling and Cognitive Behavioral Therapy

Improving psychosocial functioning along with psychotherapy tends to accompany seizure remission. Psychotherapy must involve the patients' family and any group or agency involved. Not only can this improve the patient's quality of life, but also compliance to AEDs.

c) Re-evaluation of the Anticonvulsant Regimen

For example, for treating patients with comorbid depression with epilepsy, priority should be given to AEDs that might improve mood and having antidepressant and attention-enhancing efficacy and reduce anxiety and suicidal tendencies. Some AEDs with anti-glutamatergic and sertoninergic properties may confer antidepressant, mood stabilizing and thymoleptic effects [24]. AEDs with serotonergic properties will improve mood and reduce the anxiety risk, because they exert effects similar to antidepressants (i.e. selective serotonin reuptake inhibitors or SSRIs), whereas AEDs that lack serotonergic mechanisms would not be effective in improving mood or reduction of anxiety and suicidality. Sedating drugs have anxiolytic, anti-manic and sleep-promoting benefits.

In randomized, double-blind, open-label, prospective, multicenter and clinical trials, LTG (as monotherapy and adjunctive therapy), VPA and CBZ were proved to be effective in improvement of depressive symptoms of patients with epilepsy independent of its anticonvulsant efficacy.LTG also possesses an influence on noradrenaline receptors. LTG diminishes depression, mania and has mood stabilizing effect as well as improved energy and social function besides its anti-glutamatergic activitly and serotonergic properties [136]. VPA has antidepressant. VPA is effective as mood stabilizer and in treatment of mania [139]. Although CBZ is structurally similar to the tricyclic antidepressant imipramine, it does not have antidepressant effects. CBZ can stabilize mood in bipolar disorder. CBZ effectively treats mania, impulse-control disorders, borderline personality disorder with aggression and episodic dyscontrol syndrome [144]. Stimulant effects on some aspects of psychomotor unctioning as well as improved feelings of alertness are noted with OXC [122]. PB, VGB, TGB and TPM are not recommended in the presence of depression with epilepsy. PHT is used in treatment of mania [145]. GBP [124], PGB [65], and TGB [146] have anxiolytic benefits in patients with epilepsy and anxiety. GBP and PGB improve the sense of well-being, anxiety, and insomnia and mood dysfunction independant of seizure reduction because of their sedative effect [65].TGB may improve mood and can be used in treatment of mania. TGB improves the sense of well-being, anxiety, and insomnia and can be used for treatment of anxiety [146]. In some patients, PB possesses anxiolytic, sedative hypnotic, and mood stabilizing properties. LEV but not VGB, TPM or ETX is recommended in the presence of psychosis with epilepsy. In few studies, TPM was reported to reduce aggression and obsessive symptoms which may be explained by the improvement of prefrontal brain function in epilepsy [119,125]. LTG, FBM and LEV are not recommended in the presence of anxiety with epilepsy. CBZ, OXC, VPA and LTG could be regarded as drugs with anti-suicidal properties because they all improve cognitive function and mood in epileptic patient, and possess serotonergic mechanisms of action.

d) Pharmacotherapy and other Therapeutic Modalities for Psychiatric Symptomatologies and Disorders Comorbid with Epilepsy

i) Treatment of Comorbid Depression and Epilepsy

Decreased serotonergic, noradrenergic, and GABAergic functions have been identified as pivotal pathogenic mechanisms of depression and have been the basis for antidepressant pharmacologic treatments. The efficacy of antidepressants to treat depression in patients with epilepsy has scant substantiation in the literature, but the data that do exist appear very encouraging. Selective serotonin reuptake inhibitors (SSRIs) such as citalopram (due to its lack of drug interactions), fluoxetine, fluvoxamine, sertraline, and paroxetine appear to have the lowest risk of seizure induction and are particularly recommended as first-line treatments [147]. Multireceptor-active compounds [such as nefazodone (5-hydroxytryptamine-2 antagonist), venlafaxine (combined serotonin-norepinephrine reuptake inhibitor)], monoamine oxidase inhibitors (MAOIs) [as mirtazapine (noradrenergic antidepressant) and tricyclic antidepressants (TCAs) (as amitriptyline, nortriptyline, imipramine, desipramine and doxepin)] can be used as second-line drugs but special caution is required for potential interactions with enzyme-inducing AEDs. Blumer [147] frequently used the TCA imipramine for more refractory cases. In the retrospective study done by Ojemann et al. [148], the authors observed that depressive symptoms decreased by 89%, and seizure frequency improved in 79% with TCA doxepin. In a double-blind placebo-controlled study done by Robertson and Trimble [149] using amitriptyline and nomifensine, the authors observed improvement of all patients to some degree and up to 65% improvement with increasing the dose of the antidepressants. In the study of Favale et al. [150], the authors used fluoxetine to treat 17 patients with epilepsy and symptoms of depression. The authors observed complete remission of seizure activity in 6 patients, with the remaining patients having a 30% reduction in seizure frequency and no increase in CBZ levels was observed during the study.

The most important concerns while chosing an antidepressant to treat a patient with epilepsy and depression,include:*a)* the epileptogenic potential (or proconvulsant effect), *b)* the drug-drug interaction with reduction of seizure threshold or augmentation of the a particular adverse effect of an AED, and *c)* the adverse side effects of antidepressant drug [151]. The SSRIs (fluoxetine, paroxetine, sertraline, fluvoxamine, citalopram) and the serotonin noradrenaline receptor inhibitors (SNRI) venlafaxine are the drugs of choice for patients with comorbid depression and epilepsy. They have an overall seizure induction potential of between 0.10% and 0.26% [152]. The rate can be higher in overdosage. SSRIs appear to be relatively safe, especially considering the aforementioned rate of spontaneous seizure occurrence (0.086%). Fluoxetine, however, may cause more seizure induction than do other SSRIs. Few data are available regarding seizure induction by MAOIs as mirtazapine and reboxetine. The TCAs have an overall seizure induction potential of 0.1–4.0% [153]. It has been found that TCA levels exceeding the therapeutic range were associated with seizure induction [154]. Amitriptyline and imipramine have a seizure induction potential (approximately 0.1–0.6%) that is documented to be higher than that of their respective metabolites nortriptyline and desipramine (approximately 0.1%). However, in overdose, the incidence of seizures with the metabolites increases to 22.0% for desipramine and 17.9% for nortriptyline [151-153]. Bupropion (noradrenergic-dopaminergic compound), maprotiline, amoxapine (tetracyclic antidepressants) and clomipramine (a tricyclic antidepressant), and neuroleptics have the greatest seizure risk as they lower seizure threshold and should be avoided [147-154].

Both antiepileptic and antidepressants drugs undergo hepatic biotransformation by the hepatic microsomal cytochrome P450 oxidases (3A4, 1A2, 2C19, 2C9, and, possibly, 2B6) [155] and also influence the 2D6 cytochrome. Antidepressants and antiepileptic drugscan influence these enzymes by inducing or inhibiting them. The serum levels of AED that act as a substrate for the cytochrome may be decreased if an inducing antidepressant drug is added, with decreasing of seizure threshold while enzyme inhibitor may decrease the metabolism of AEDs, thus increasing toxicity from the AED.

The serotonin syndrome is a rare disorder that may result from drug interactions between AEDs of serotonergic properties and SSRIs. It is caused by excessive serotoninergic stimulation, symptoms include: restlessness, myoclonus, hyperthermia, convulsions and possibly death) [156]. Furthermore, PHT and CBZ may hypothetically lower mirtazapine levels, and cases of agranulocytosis or neutropenia have been associated with this agent. Combining it with another bone marrow–suppressing drug, such as CBZ, should be avoided [157].

One challenging question has to be addressed while evaluating comorbid depression and epilepsy. *This question Is determining the epileptogenic potential of each antidepressant drug is difficult?.* The answer is Yes, determining the epileptogenic potential of each antidepressant drug is difficult and extremely complex for the following reasons: *1)* the extent of concordance between animal and clinical trials, for example: maprotiline in animal studies was thought to be relatively safe but, when marketed, was found to be one of the more epileptogenic antidepressant compounds [157], *2)* how adequate are the pharmacological methodologies, *3)* the lack of investigational, clinical or follow up studies that demonstrate the therapeutic efficacy of antidepressant drugs with epilepsy, *4)* Considering the rate of natural occurrence of a seizure in the general population, the overall incidence of a first seizure was calculated to be approximately 0.086% [158], thus any drug considered to be a severe risk for seizure induction would, therefore, have to demonstrate a rate higher than the rate of spontaneousoccurrence.

Some considerations have to be taken to overcome such obstacles as follow: *1)* Careful followup of the serum levels of antiepileptic and antidepressants (drug-drug interaction) have to be undertaken while treating comorbid depression with epilepsy. The AEDs most commonly responsible for interactions with antidepressants are the cytochrome-inducing drugs (as CBZ, PHT and PB)and the inhibitory agents(as VPA) [159,160]. Clinically significant elevations of these AEDs have been observed when used in combination with fluoxetine and thus fluoxetine should not be used in combination with CBZ, PHT, or PB, or, at the least, serum monitoring is required.TCAs are metabolized via the 2D6 cytochrome and thus patients with congenital deficiencies of this enzyme may exhibit elevation of serum levels, *2)* Gradual escalation in antidepressant dosages is recommended while treating comorbid depression and epilepsy as rapidity of dosage escalation is other factor for increase in seizure frequency with antidepressants, and *3)* Chosing other treatment modalities for treatment of severe, treatment-resistant, or psychotic depression and independent of effect on seizure frequency which include: neuroleptics [157], electroconvulsive therapy (ECT) [161] and vagus nerve stimulation (VNS) [162]

ii) Treatment of Comorbid Psychosis and Epilepsy

Chronic inter-ictal psychosis requires the use of chronic therapy with antipsychotic drugs to obtain remission of psychotic symptoms. While chosing an antipsychotic to treat a patient with epilepsy and psychosis, the epileptogenic potential, the drug-drug interaction and the adverse side effects of the antipsychotic drug should be considered. The atypical antipsychotic agents have largely replaced their older relatives, except in more acute circumstances (e.g., postictal psychosis) in which parenteral forms are required. For example, for emergent symptoms, intravenous haloperidol can be used. Halopridol, one of the most common tradition or typical antipsychotics, is easy to administer and seems to have fewer extrapyramidal side effects than the oral preparation, although the evidence is sparse [163]. After controllong the emergent symptoms, the dosage of haloperidol will then be gradually reduced usually over the next several weeks, as tolerated by the patient. This will be followed by a subsequent shift to a more atypical neuroleptic.

The typical neuroleptics antipsychotic drugs [as phenothiazines (chlorpromazine, fluphenazine, trifluoperazine, perphenazine and thioridazine), butyrophenones (haloperidol), thioxanthenes (thiothixene), dihydroindolones (molindone) and dibenzoxazepines (loxapine)]function isalmost exclusively depending on their affinity for blocking the dopamine D2 receptor site. In contrast, the atypical antipsychotics (as clozapine, risperidone, olanzapine, and quetiapine) additionally block other dopamine subtypes and serotonin receptors. The significantly decreased rate of extrapyramidal side effects and tardive dyskinesia associated with the atypical agents probably stems from these unique factors [164]. All antipsychotic medications decrease the seizure threshold to varying degrees [165,166]. Clozapine has greater affinity toD1 than D2 and increased D3 and D4 antagonism. It also has effect on serotonin receptors, however, its dose-dependent lowering effect on the seizure threshold has greatly limited its utility in treating epilepsy patients in addition to its adverse side effects which include: agranulocytosis, with an incidence of 1% in the first year and a maximal risk in the initial 4 to 18 weeks of treatment [166]. The antipsychotics of choice on the basis ofless epileptogenic potentials and of the less side effect profiles are risperidone, olanzapine and quetiapine. Like clozapine, risperidone, olanzapine and quetiapine have potent serotoninergic activity and sparing effects on the nigrostriatal dopaminergic neurons, with much lower incidence of extrapyramidal side effects, tardive dyskinesia, and malignant neuroleptic syndrome than with typical antipsychotics [164]. However, they are not free of side effects as follow: risperidone may cause QT interval prolongation, olanzapine may induce hepatic transaminase enzyme elevations especially in the first few weeks) which eventually may normalize and quetiapine may produce lens changes that may require intermittent ocular examinations.

For typical antipsychotics with highest risk of seizure induction;loxapine and chlorpromazine, while fluphenazine, thioridazine, perphenazine and trifluoperazine, have an intermediate range of less than 1.0–1.2%. Haloperidol, molindone and pimozide have the least seizure-induction activity. The possible mechanisms by which antipsychotics lower the seizure threshold include disruption of the dopaminergic-cholinergic balance and depletion of GABA. Seizure potential is dose-related, so high-dose therapy and rapid upward dose titration should be avoided.

Most antipsychotics are metabolized by the 2D6 and CYP3A subfamilies of the cytochrome P450 system. Thus, drug-drug interaction is a significant possibility. PB and CBZ can lower serum levels of antipsychotics as risperidone, olanzapine and haloperidol (as much as 50–60%). In addition, coadministration of CBZ and antipsychotic may aggravate psychosis and may result in neuroleptic malignant syndrome [159].

Antipsychotics can also be used to treat epilepsy with the following comorbid psychiatric problems: 1) severe or medication resistant depression, psychotic depression, psychosis, 2) PIP: As progression from postictal to interictal psychosis is not uncommon. In about 15% of patients, interictal psychotic symptoms may occur after an episode of PIP, thus increased awareness and prompt treatment of PIP may inhibit or prevent development of some instances of interictal psychosis, 3) chronic inter-ictal psychosis, 4) aggression, 5) some personality disorders.

iii) Treatment of Comorbid Bipolar Affective Disorder and Epilepsy

Although, lithium is considered pro-convulsant but has been used safely in patients with epilepsy and bipolar affective disorder and may augment the effect of some AEDs. However, it should be used with caution in patients with epilepsy. An encephalopathy was rarely reported when lithium was used in combination with CBZ [167].

iv) Treatment of Comorbid Anxiety and Behavioral Dyscontrol Syndrome and Epilepsy

Anxiety and behavioral dyscontrol can be a significant problem in patients with depressive disorder and comorbid epilepsy. In particular, overarousal and dysfunction of the serotonin system have been implicated as frequent primary factors. Pregabalin (PGB) has proven anxiolytic property and has shown to be effective and safe treatment for generalized anxiety disorder and thus can be used for treatment ofcomorbid anxiety and behavioral dyscontrol with epilepsy. Buspirone is a non-benzodiazepine that currently is marketed as an anti-anxiety agent. It appears to exert partial agonist activity at the 5-hydroxy-tryptamine-1A receptor. At low dosages, it has been found to be useful for ameliorating aggression. It does not appear to interact with anticonvulsants.However, in animal models, buspirone has been shown to be proconvulsant [168]. In addition, one case report cites a patient who sustained a seizure after an overdose of buspirone [169].

Table 5. The biopsychosocial approach to manage patients with epilepsy and inter-ictal behavioral abnormalities

1. *Optimizing seizure control*
2. *Psychotherapy, counseling and cognitive behavioral therapy*
3. *Re-evaluation of the anticonvulsant regimen* with priority should be given to AEDs that have mood stabilizing, thymoleptic, antidepressant, anxiolytic, attention-enhancing efficacy and reducing suicidal tendenciesas LTG, VPA, CBZ and OXC (but notPB, VGB, TGB or TPM) for depression, GBP, PGB and TGB (but not LTG, FBM, LEV, PB or Benzodiazepines) for anxiety and LEV (but not VGB, TPM, ETX) for psychosis, PHT, CBZ, OXC and TGB for mania, TPM for obsession, CBZ, OXC, VPA and LTG for suicide thoughts and attempts.
4. *Pharmacotherapy for psychiatric symptomatologies and disorders comorbid with epilepsy*
For the prescribed drugs, caution should be paid to:
a) the epileptogenic potential (or proconvulsants)
b) the drug-drug interaction with reduction of seizure threshold due to reduction of the serum level of utilized AEDs
c) augmentation of the particular adverse effect of an AED
d) The adverse side effects of psychotropic drugs.
For depression:
First line-choice drugs (drugs with lowest risk): The SSRIs (fluoxetine, paroxetine, sertraline, fluvoxamine, citalopram) and the serotonin noradrenaline receptor inhibitors (SNRI) venlafaxine
Second line-choice drugs (Drugs with intermediate risk): Multireceptor-active compounds [as nefazodone (5-hydroxytryptamine-2 antagonist), monoamine oxidase inhibitors (MAOIs) [as mirtazapine (noradrenergic antidepressant) and tricyclic antidepressants (TCAs) (as amitriptyline, nortriptyline, imipramine, desipramine and doxepin) can be used as second-line drugs
Drugs to be avoided (Drugs with highest risk): Bupropion (noradrenergic-dopaminergic compound), maprotiline, amoxapine (tetracyclic antidepressants) and clomipramine (a tricyclic antidepressant), and some neuroleptics
For psychosis:
Emergency psychotic manifestations: parenteral halopridol
*First line-choice drugs (drugs with lowest risk):*Haloperidol, molindone, pimozide, Risperidone, quetiapine and olanzapine
Second line-choice drugs (Drugs with intermediate risk): Fluphenazine, thioridazine, perphenazine and trifluoperazine
Drugs to be avoided (Drugs with highest risk): Loxapine and chlorpromazine and clozapine
For bipolar affective disorder:
Lithium
For neurosis, anxiety and behavioral dyscontrol syndrome:
Pregabalin and gabapentin
For attention deficit hyperactive disorders (ADHD):
Methylphenidate

Beta-blockers asnadolol and propranolol may be useful for modulating overstimulation and to treat aggression in patients with epilepsy [170]. The beta-blockers decrease hyperarousal, restlessness, and tension. They decrease anxiety and cause little cognitive compromise. Nadolol works peripherally, whereas propranolol is more lipophilic and exerts more CNS effects. Both medications, especially propranolol, may require titration to obtain an effective dosage. However, propranolol has been noted to be associated with seizure activity in overdosage.However, in some animal models, it appears to increase the seizure threshold [171]. In addition, depression is a rare side effect of propranolol [170].

Benzodiazepines and barbiturates should not be used as anxiolytics in people with epilepsy, because of the danger of dependence and the potential for withdrawal seizures.

v) Treatment of Comorbid ADHD and Epilepsy

In preliminary studies, methylphenidate has been found effective against adult ADHD with no adverse effects on seizure severity and frequency [172]. Methylphenidate has a proven efficacy in treatment of children with isolated ADHD and comorbid ADHD and epilepsy in children [49]. However, few studies in the pediatric population reported seizure aggravation in children with uncontrolled epilepsy with methylphenidate [173]. Amphetamines which are the mainstay of therapy for patients displaying impulsivity, distractibility, and motor overactivity in the constellation of a diagnosis of ADHD, do not seem to be the drug of choice in adult population with ADHD and epilepsy as impulsivity, distractibility, and motor overactivity are less prominent symptomatology in adult ADHD comorbid with epilepsy. In addition, it can be associated with seizure activity.

Conclusion

Psychiatric symptomatologies and disorders are frequent comorbidities in patients with epilepsy and have significant impact on the medical management, compliance to medications and quality of life. Although the mechanisms of psychiatric comorbidities with epilepsy are complex and poorly understood, however, both epilepsy itself as well as antiepileptic medications, are contributed. This should attract attention of scientests interested in the field of epilepsy towards better understanding of the exact pathophysiologic mechanisms of psychiatric comorbidities with epilepsy. This will move management of patients towards a comprehensive neuropsychobiological approach (pharmacological and non-pharmacological approaches) which focuses on the whole person rather than simply on the disease process.

References

[1] Hauser WA. Incidence and prevalence. In: Engel J, Pedley TA, eds. Epilepsy: a comprehensive textbook. Philadelphia: *Lippincott-Raven* 1997;47-57.

[2] Osuntokun BO. Epilepsy in the African continent. In: Peny JK (ed.). *Epilepsy: The eighth international symposium PP*. New York, Ravan Press, 1977;365–78.

[3] Shawki A. Etiological and clinical presentation of epilepsy in Upper Egypt. M.D. Thesis in Neurology. Faculty of Medicine, Assiut University. 1995.

[4] Engel J Jr. Update on surgical treatment of the epilepsies. Summary of the Second International Palm Desert Conference on the Surgical Treatment of the Epilepsies (1992). *Neurology*. 1993;43(8):1612-7.

[5] Blanchet P, Frommer GP. Mood change preceding epileptic seizures. *J Nerv Ment Dis* 1986;174(8):471–6.

[6] Biraben A, Taussig D, Thomas P, Even C, Vignal JP, Scarabin JM, Chauvel P. Fear as the main feature of epileptic seizures. *J Neurol Neurosurg Psychiatry* 2001;70(2): 186–91.

[7] Kanner AM, Stagno S, Kotagal P. Postictal psychiatric events during prolonged video-electroencephalographic monitoring studies. *Arch Neurol* 1996;53(3):258-63.

[8] Kanemoto K, Kawasaki J, Mori E. Violence and epilepsy: a close relation between violence and postictal psychosis. *Epilepsia* 1999;40(1):107-9.

[9] Kobau R, Gilliam F, Thurman DJ. Prevalence of self-reported epilepsy or seizure disorder and its associations with self-reported depression and anxiety: results from the 2004 HealthStyles Survey. *Epilepsia* 2006;47(11):1915-21.

[10] Mula M. The clinical spectrum of bipolar symptoms in epilepsy: a critical reappraisal. *Postgrad Med.* 2010;122(4):17-23.

[11] Beyenburg S, Mitchell AJ, Schmidt D, Elger CE, Reuber M. Anxiety in patients with epilepsy: systematic review and suggestions for clinical management. *Epilepsy Behav* 2005;7(2):161-71.

[12] Dongier S. Statistical study of clinical and electroencephalographic manifestations of 536 psychotic episodes occurring in 516 epileptics between clinical seizures. *Epilepsia* 1959;1:117-42.

[13] Ertekin BA, Kulaksizoğlu IB, Ertekin E, Gürses C, Bebek N, Gökyiğit A, Baykan B. A comparative study of obsessive-compulsive disorder and other psychiatric comorbidities in patients with temporal lobe epilepsy and idiopathic generalized epilepsy. *Epilepsy Behav* 2009;14(4):634-9.

[14] Koneski JA, Casella EB. Attention deficit and hyperactivity disorder in people with epilepsy: diagnosis and implications to the treatment. *Arq Neuropsiquiatr.* 2010;68(1):107-14.

[15] Lopez-Rodriguez F, Altshuler L, Kay J, Delarhim S, Mendez M, Engel J Jr. Personality disorders among medically refractory epileptic patients. *J Neuropsychiatry Clin Neurosci* 1999;11(4):464–9.

[16] van Elst LT, Woermann FG, Lemieux L, Thompson PJ, Trimble MR. Affective aggression in patients with temporal lobe epilepsy, A quantitative MRI study of the amygdala. *Brain* 2000;123(Pt 2):234-43.

[17] Christensen J, Vestergaard M, Mortensen PB, Sidenius P, Agerbo E. Epilepsy and risk of suicide: a population-based case-control study. *Lancet Neurol* 2007;6(8):693-8.

[18] Perrine K, Hermann BP, Meador KJ, Vickrey BG, Cramer JA, Hays RD. The relationship of neuropsychological functioning to quality of life in epilepsy. *Arch Neurol* 1995;52(10):997-1003.

[19] Mrabet H, Mrabet A, Zouari B, Ghachem R. Health-related quality of life of people with epilepsy compared with a general reference population: a Tunisian study. *Epilepsia* 2004;45(7):838–43.

[20] Pennell PB, Thompson P. Gender-specific psychosocial impact of living with epilepsy. *Epilepsy Behav* 2009;15 (Suppl 1):S20-5.

[21] Engel J, Wilson C, Lopez-Rodriguez F. Limbic connectivity: anatomical substrates of behavioural disturbances in epilepsy. In: Trimble M, Schmitz B, eds. *The neuropsychiatry of epilepsy.* Cambridge: Cambridge University Press 2002:18–37.
[22] Helmstaedter C. Behavioral aspects of frontal lobe epilepsy. *Epilepsy Behav* 2001;2(5):384–95.
[23] Broicher S, Kuchukhidze G, Grunwald T, Krämer G, Kurthen M, Trinka E, Jokeit H. Association between structural abnormalities and fMRI response in the amygdala in patients with temporal lobe epilepsy. *Seizure* 2010;19(7):426-31.
[24] Ketter TA, Post RM, Theodore WH. Positive and negative psychiatric effects of antiepileptic drugs in patients with seizure disorders. *Neurology* 1999;53(Suppl 2): S53–67.
[25] Nadkarni S, Devinsky O. Psychotropic Effects of Antiepileptic Drugs. *Epilepsy* Current 2005;5(5):176-81.
[26] Mula M, Marotta AE, Monaco F. Epilepsy and bipolar disorders. *Expert Rev Neurother.* 2010;10(1):13-23.
[27] Mazza M, Di Nicola M, Della Marca G, Janiri L, Bria P, Mazza S. Bipolar disorder and epilepsy: a bidirectional relation? Neurobiological underpinnings, current hypotheses, and future research directions. *Neuroscientist.* 2007;13(4):392-404.
[28] Dhir A. Novel discoveries in understanding the complexities of epilepsy and major depression. *Expert Opin Ther Targets.* 2010;14(1):109-15.
[29] Kanner AM. Depression and epilepsy: A bidirectional relation? *Epilepsia.* 2011;52 (Suppl 1):21-7.
[30] Manchanda R, Freeland A, Schaefer B, McLachlan RS, Blume WT. Auras, seizure focus, and psychiatric disorders. *Neuropsychiatry Neuropsychol Behav Neurol* 2000;13(1):13-9.
[31] Alemayehu S, Bergey GK, Barry E, Krumholz A, Wolf A, Fleming CP, Frear EJ Jr Panic attacks as ictal manifestations of parietal lobe seizures. *Epilepsia* 1995;36(8):824–30.
[32] Kanner AM. Recognition of the Various Expressions of Anxiety, Psychosis and Aggression in Epilepsy. *Epilepsia* 2004;45(Suppl 2):22-7.
[33] So NK, Savard G, Andermann F, Olivier A, Quesney LF. Acute postictal psychosis: a stereo EEG study. *Epilepsia.* 1990;31(2):188-93.
[34] Kanner AM, Trimble M, Schmitz B. Postictal affective episodes. *Epilepsy Behav.* 2010 Oct;19(2):156-8.
[35] Ettinger A, Reed M, Cramer J. Depression and comorbidity in community-based patients with epilepsy or asthma. *Neurology* 2004;63(6):1008-14.
[36] Mensah SA, Beavis JM, Thapar AK. The presence and clinical implications of depression in a community population of adults with epilepsy. *Epilepsy Behav* 2006;8(1):213-9.
[37] Weissman MM, Bland R, Joyce PR, Newman S, Wells JE, Wittchen HU. Sex differences in rates of depression: Cross-national perspectives. *J Affect Disord* 1993;29(2-3):77–84.
[38] Mendez MF, Cummings JL, Benson DF. Depression in epilepsy. Significance and phenomenology. *Arch Neurology* 1986;43(8):766-70.

[39] Glosser G, Zwil AS, Glosser DS, O'Connor MJ, Sperling MR.Psychiatric aspects of temporal lobe epilepsy before and after anterior temporal lobectomy. *J Neurol Neurosurg Psychiatry* 2000;68(1):53–8.

[40] Karouni M, Arulthas S, Larsson PG, Rytter E, Johannessen SI, Landmark CJ. Psychiatric comorbidity in patients with epilepsy: a population-based study. *Eur J Clin Pharmacol* 2010;66(11):1151-60.

[41] Weissman MM, Bland RC, Canino GJ, Faravelli C, Greenwald S, Hwu H, Joyce PR, Karam EG, Lee C, Lellouch J, Lépine J, Newman SC, Rubio-Stipec M, Wells JE, Wickramaratne PJ, Wittchen H, Yeh E. Cross-National Epidemiology of Major Depression and Bipolar Disorder. *JAMA* 1996;276(4):293-9.

[42] Ettinger AB, Reed ML, Goldberg JF, Hirschfeld RM. Prevalence of bipolar symptoms in epilepsy vs other chronic health disorders. *Neurology.* 2005;65(4):535-40.

[43] Blumer D. Dysphoric disorders and paroxysmal affects: recognition and treatment of epilepsy-related psychiatric disorders. *Harv Rev Psychiatry*2000 ;8(1):8-17.

[44] Kessler RC, McGonagle KA, Zhao S, Nelson CB, Hughes M, Eshleman S, Wittchen HU, Kendler KS. Lifetime and 12-month prevalence of DSM-III-R psychiatric disorders in the United States. Results from the National Comorbidity Survey. *Arch Gen Psychiatry* 1994;51(1):8-19.

[45] Fullana MA, Vilagut G, Rojas-Farreras S, Mataix-Cols D, de Graaf R, Demyttenaere K, Haro JM, de Girolamo G, Lépine JP, Matschinger H, Alonso J; ESEMeD/MHEDEA 2000 investigators. Obsessive-compulsive symptom dimensions in the general population: results from an epidemiological study in six European countries. *J Affect Disord* 2010;124(3):291-9.

[46] Allen IM. Forced thinking as part of the epileptic attack. *NZ Med J*1952;51(282):86–95.

[47] Waxman SG, Geschwind N. The interictal behavior syndrome of temporal lobe epilepsy. *Arch Gen* Psychiatry 1976;32(12):1580–6.

[48] Geschwind N (1983) *Pathogenesis of behaviour change in temporal lobe epilepsy.* In: Ward AA Jr, Penry JK, Purpura DP, eds. Epilepsy. New York: Raven Press 355–70.

[49] Kaufmann R, Goldberg-Stern H, Shuper A. Attention-deficit disorders and epilepsy in childhood: incidence, causative relations and treatment possibilities *J Child Neurol* 2009;24(6):727-33.

[50] Faraone SV, Biederman J, Spencer T, Wilens T, Seidman LJ, Mick E, Doyle AE. Attention-deficit/hyperactivity disorder in adults: an overview. *Biological Psychiatry* 2000;48(1):9-20.

[51] Swinkels WA, Duijsens IJ, Spinhoven P. Personality disorder traits in patients with epilepsy. *Seizure* 2003;12(8):587-94.

[52] Torgersen S, Kringlen E, Cramer V. The prevalence of personality disorders in a community sample. *Arch Gen Psychiatry* 2001;58(6):590-6.

[53] Pizzi AM, Chapin JS, Tesar GE, Busch RM. Comparison of personality traits in patients with frontal and temporal lobe epilepsies. *Epilepsy Behav* 2009;15(2):225-9.

[54] Wilson SJ, Wrench JM, McIntosh AM, Bladin PF, Berkovic SF. Personality development in the context of intractable epilepsy. *Arch Neurol* 2009;66(1):68-72.

[55] de Araújo Filho GM, Jackowski AP, Lin K, Guaranha MS, Guilhoto LM, da Silva HH, Caboclo LO, Júnior HC, Bressan RA, Yacubian EM Personality traits related to juvenile myoclonic epilepsy: MRI reveals prefrontal abnormalities through a voxel-based morphometry study. *Epilepsy Behav* 2009;15(2):202-7.

[56] Tarulli A, Devinsky O, Alper K. Progression of postictal to interictal psychosis. *Epilepsia* 2001;42(11):1468-71.
[57] Kumari V, Ffytche DH, Williams SCR, Gray JA. Personality predicts brain responses to cognitive demands. *J Neurosci* 2004;24:10636–41.
[58] Jallon P. Mortality in patients with epilepsy. *Current Opinion in Neurology* 2004;17(2):141-146.
[59] Christensen J, Vestergaard M, Mortensen PB, Sidenius P, Agerbo E. Epilepsy and risk of suicide: a population-based case-control study. *Lancet Neurol* 2007;6(8):693-698.
[60] Bell GS, Gaitatzis A, Bell CL, Johnson AL, Sander JW. Suicide in people with epilepsy: how great is the risk?.*Epilepsia* 2009;50(8):1933-42.
[61] Bolton JM, Robinson J.Population-attributable fractions of Axis I and Axis II mental disorders for suicide attempts: findings from a representative sample of the adult, noninstitutionalized US population. *Am J Public Health* 2010;100(12):2473-480.
[62] Pompili M, Girardi P, Tatarelli R. Death from suicide versus mortality from epilepsy in the epilepsies: a meta-analysis. *Epilepsy Behav* 2006;9(4):641-8.
[63] Jones JE, Hermann BP, Barry JJ, Gilliam FG, Kanner AM, Meador KJ. Rates and risk factors for suicide, suicidal ideation, and suicide attempts in chronic epilepsy. *Epilepsy Behav* 2003;4(Suppl 3):S31-38.
[64] Hesdorffer DC, HauserWA, Olafsson E, Ludvigsson P, Kjartansson O.Depression and suicidal attempt as risk factor for incidental unprovoked seizures. *Ann Neurol* 2006;59(1):35–41.
[65] Betts T. Psychiatric disorder in epilepsy. In: Duncan JS, Sisodiya SM, Smalls JE, eds. Epilepsy 2001. From science to patient. Oxford:*International League Against Epilepsy* 2001:257–60.
[66] Quiske A, Helmstaedter C, Lux S, Elger CE. Depression in patients with temporal lobe epilepsy is related to mesial temporal sclerosis. *Epilepsy Res* 2000;39(2):121-5.
[67] Gilliam FG, Maton BM, Martin RC, Sawrie SM, Faught RE, Hugg JW, Viikinsalo M, Kuzniecky RI. Hippocampal 1H-MRSI correlates with severity of depression symptoms in temporal lobe epilepsy.*Neurology* 2007;68(5):364-8.
[68] Swinkels WAM, Boas WVE, Kuyk J, Dyck RV, Spinhoven P. Inter-ictalpsychopathology in temporal lobe epilepsy (TLE) and extra-temporal lobe epilepsy. *Epilepsia* 2006;47(12):2092-03.
[69] Satishchandra P, Krishnamoorthy ES, van Elst LT. Mesial temporal structures and comorbid anxiety in refractory partial epilepsy. *J Neuropsychiatry Clin Neurosci* 2003;15(4):450–2.
[70] Isaacs KL, Philbeck JW, Barr WB, Devinsky O, Alper K. Obsessive-compulsive symptoms in patients with temporal lobe epilepsy.*Epilepsy Behavior* 2004;5(4):569-74.
[71] Amo C, Santiuste M, Maestú F, Fernández A, Egatz R, González-Hidalgo M, Saldaña C, Sáiz A, Ortiz T. Temporal lobe seizure recorded by magnetoencephalography: case report. *Arq Neuropsiquiatr* 2004;62(3A):737-40.
[72] Mendez MF, Engebrit B, Doss R, Grau R. The relationship of epileptic auras and psychological attributes. *J Neuropsychiatry Clin Neurosci* 1996;8(3):287-92.
[73] Mellers JD, Adachi N, Takei N, Cluckie A, Toone BK, Lishman WA. SPET study of verbal fluency in schizophrenia and epilepsy. *Br J Psychiatry*1998;173:69-74.
[74] Perez MM, Trimble MR. Epileptic psychosis--diagnostic comparison with process schizophrenia. *Br J Psychiatry1980*;137:245-9.

[75] Delgado-Escueta AV, Swartz BE, Walsh GO, Chauvel P, Bancaud J, Broglin D. Frontal lobe seizures and epilepsies in neurobehavioraldisorders. *Advances in Neurology* 1991;55:317–240.

[76] Powell AL, Yudd A, Zee P, Mandelbaum DE. Attention deficithyperactivity disorder associated with orbitofrontal epilepsy in a father and a son. Neuropsychiatry, *Neuropsychology, and Behavioral Neurology* 1997;10(2):151-4.

[77] Miller K, Kłopotowski T, Rościszewska D. Suicide attempts in epileptic patients during the years 1990-92. Analysis of patients in the Regional Poison Control Center in Sosnowiec. *Psychiatr Pol.* 1997;31(6):667-675.

[78] Nilsson L, Ahlbom A, Farahmand BY, Asberg M, Tomson T. Riskfactors for suicide in epilepsy: a case control study. *Epilepsia*2002;43(6):644–651.

[79] Kalinin VV, Polyanskiy DA. Gender differences in risk factors of suicidal behavior in epilepsy *Epilepsy Behav* 2005;6(3):424-429.

[80] Verrotti A, Cicconetti A, Scorrano B, De Berardis D, Cotellessa C, Chiarelli F, Ferro FM. Epilepsy and suicide: pathogenesis, risk factors, and prevention. Neuropsychiatr *Dis Treat* 2008;4(2):365-70.

[81] Cornaggia CM, Massimiliano Beghi, Milena Provenzi, Ettore Beghi. Correlation between Cognition and Behavior in Epilepsy. *Epilepsia* 2006;47(Suppl 2):34–3.

[82] Bell GS, Sander JW. Suicide and epilepsy. *Curr Opin Neurol* 2009;22(2):174-8.

[83] Hamed SA. Neuronal Plasticity: Implications in Epilepsy Progression and Management. *Drug Develop Res* 2007;68(8):498-511.

[84] Engel J, Shewmon DA. Impact of the kindling phenomenon on clinical epileptology. In: Morrell F, ed. *Kindling and synaptic plasticity: the legancy of graham Goddard.* Cambridge 1991;195–210.

[85] Elst LT, Groffmann M, Ebert D, Schulze-Bonhage A. Amygdala volume loss in patients with dysphoric disorder of epilepsy. *Epilepsy Behav* 2009;16(1):105-12.

[86] Drevets WC. Functional neuroimaging studies of depression: the anatomy of melancholia. *Annu Rev Med* 1998;49:341-61.

[87] Steriade M. Corticothalamic resonance, states of vigilance and mentation. *Neuroscience* 2000;101(2):243–76.

[88] Bremner JD, Narayan M, Anderson ER, Staib LH, Miller HL, Charney DS. Hippocampal volume reduction in major depression. *Am J Psychiatry* 2000;157(1): 115-8.

[89] Richardson EJ, Griffith HR, Martin RC, Paige AL, Stewart CC, Jones J, Hermann BP, Seidenberg M. Structural and functional neuroimaging correlates of depression in temporal lobe epilepsy. *Epilepsy Behav* 2007;10(2):242-9.

[90] Shih JJ, Weisend MP, Sanders JA, Lee RR. Magnetoencephalographic and Magnetic Resonance Spectroscopy Evidence of Regional Functional Abnormality in Mesial Temporal Lobe Epilepsy. *Brain Topogr.* 2011;23(4):368-74.

[91] Ryvlin P, Philippon B, Cinotti L, Froment JC, Le Bars D, Mauguière F. Functional neuroimaging strategy in temporal lobe epilepsy: a comparative study of 18FDG-PET and 99mTc-HMPAO-SPECT. *Ann Neurol* 1992;31(6):650-6.

[92] Sah P, Faber ES, Lopez De Armentia M, Power J. The amygdaloid complex: Anatomy and physiology. *Physoil Rev* 2003;83(3):803-34.

[93] Malizia AL. What do brain imaging studies tell us about anxiety disorders? *J Psychopharmacol* 1999;13(4):372–8.

[94] Eron LD, Gruder CL. Some topics closely related to the study of abnormal behavior: aggression and fantasy. In: Reiss S et al., editors. *Abnormality: experimental and clinical approaches.* New York: Macmillan; 1977:579–638.
[95] Stuss DT, Levine B. Adult clinical neuropsychology: lessons from studies of the frontal lobes. *Annu Rev Psychol* 2002;53:401-33.
[96] Doyle AE. Executive functions in attention-deficit/hyperactivity disorder. *J Clin Psychiatry* 2006;67(Suppl 8):21–6.
[97] Zametkin A, Liotta W. The neurobiology of attention-deficit/hyperactivity disorder. *J Clin Psychiatry* 1998;59(Suppl 7):17-23.
[98] Jobe PC, Dailey JW, Wernicke JF. A noradrenergic and serotonergic hypothesis of the linkage between epilepsy and affective disorders. *Crit Rev Neurobiol* 1999;13(4): 317-56.
[99] Lydiard RB. The role of GABA in anxiety disorders. *J Clin Psychiatry* 2003;64 (Suppl 3):21–7.
[100] Hasler G, Bonwetsch R, Giovacchini G, Toczek MT, Bagic A, Luckenbaugh DA, Drevets WC, Theodore WH. 5-HTIA receptor bindingin temporal lobe epilepsy patients with and without major depression. *Biol Psychiatry* 2007;62(11):1258-64.
[101] Bortolato M, Solbrig MV. The price of seizure control: dynorphins in interictal and postictal psychosis. *Psychiat Ret* 2007;151(1-2):139-43.
[102] Krause K, Deresl SH, Krause J. Increased striatal dopamine transporter in adult patients with attention deficit hyper activity disorders, effects of methylphenidate as measured by single photon emission tomography. *Neuroscience* 2000;285(2):107-10.
[103] Bagdy G, Kecskemeti V, Riba P, Jakus R. Serotonin and epilepsy. *Neurochem* 2007;100:857–73.
[104] Richerson GB, Buchanan GF.The serotonin axis: Shared mechanisms in seizures, depression, and SUDEP. *Epilepsia.* 2011;52(Suppl 1):28-38.
[105] Forsgren L, Nystrom L. An incident case-referent study of epileptic seizures in adults. *Epilepsy Res* 1990;6(1):66–81.
[106] Baron M. Genetic linkage and bipolar affective disorder: Progress and pitfalls. *Mol Psychiatry* 1997;2(3):200-10.
[107] Hamed SA, Mohamed KA, EL-taher, AM, Hamed EA, Omar H. The Sexual and Reproductive Health in Men with Generalized Epilepsy: A Multidisciplinary Evaluation. *International Journal of Impotence Research* 2006;18(3):287-92.
[108] Kuzniecky R, Ho S, Pan J. Modulation of cerebral GABA By topiramate, lamotrigine, and gabapentin in healthy adults. *Neurology* 2002;58(3):368-72.
[109] Ried S., Mothersil I.W. Forced normalization: the clinical neurologist's view. In: Forced normalization and alternative psychoses of epilepsy. Trimble M.R., Schmttz B (ed). *Wrightson Biomedical* 1998;77-94.
[110] Tugendhaft P, Ansseau M, de Borchgrave V, Delvaux V, de Tourtchaninoff M, Dubru JM, Floris M, Foulon M, Grisar T, Hmaimess G, Legros B, Mahieu B, Ossemann M, Sadzot B, van Ruckevorsel K, Verheulpen D. Guidelines for recognition and treatment of the psychoses associated with epilepsy. *Acta neurol Belg* 2005;105(1):14-7.
[111] Fröscher W, Maier V, Laage M, Wolfersdorf M, Straub R, Rothmeier J, Steinert T, Fiaux A, Frank U, Grupp D. Folate deficiency, anticonvulsant drugs, and psychiatric morbidity. *Clin Neuropharmacol* 1995;18(2):165-82.

[112] Skarupski KA, Tangney C, Li H, Ouyang B, Evans DA, Morris MC. Longitudinal association of vitamin B-6, folate, and vitamin B-12 with depressive symptoms among older adults over time. *Am J Clin Nutr* 2010;92(2):330-5.

[113] Yanai J, Fares F, Gavish M, Greenfeld Z, Katz Y, Marcovici G, Pick CG, Rogel-Fuchs Y, Weizman A. Neural and behavioral alterations after early exposure to phenobarbital. *Neurotoxicology* 1989;10(3):543–54.

[114] Levinson DF, Devinsky O. Psychiatric adverse events during vigabatrin therapy. *Neurology* 2001;53(7):1503-11.

[115] Leppik IE, Gram L, Deaton R, Sommerville KW. Safety of tiagabine: summary of 53 trials. *Epilepsy Res* 1999;33(2-3):235-46.

[116] Cramer JA, De Rue K, Devinsky O, Edrich P, Trimble MR. A systematic review of the behavioral effects of levetiracetam in adults with epilepsy, cognitive disorders, or an anxiety disorder during clinical trials. *Epilepsy Behav* 2003;4(2):124-32.

[117] McConnell H, Snyder PJ, Duffy JD, Weilburg J, Valeriano J, Brillman J, Cress K, Cavalier J. Neuropsychiatric side effects related to felbamate. *J Neuropsychiatry Clin Neurosci* 1996;8(3):341-46.

[118] Park SP, Hwang YH, Lee HW, Suh CK, Kwon SH, Lee BI. Long-term cognitive and mood effects of zonisamide monotherapy in epilepsy patients. *Epilepsy Behav* 2008;12(1):102-8.

[119] Mula M, Trimble MR, Lhatoo SD, Sander JW. Topiramate and psychiatric adverse events in patients with epilepsy. *Epilepsia* 2003;44(5):659-63.

[120] Smith DB, Mattson RH, Cramer JA, Collins JF, Novelly RA, Craft B. Results of a nationwide Veterans Administration Cooperative Study comparing the efficacy and toxicity of carbamazepine, phenobarbital, phenytoin, and primidone. *Epilepsia* 1987;28(Suppl 3):S50-8.

[121] Nowakowska E, Kus K, Czubak A, Glowacka D, Matschay A. Some behavioural effects of carbamazepine-comparison with haloperidol. *J Physiol Pharmacol* 2007;58(2):253-64.

[122] Curran HV, Java R. Memory and psychomotor effects of oxcarbamazepine in healthy human volunteers. *Eur J Clin Pharmacol* 1993;44(6):529-33.

[123] Mecarelli O, Vicenzini E, Pulitano P, Vanacore N, Romolo FS, Di Piero V, Lenzi GL, Accornero N. Clinical, cognitive and neurophysiologic correlates of short-term treatment with carbamazepine, oxcarbazepine and levetiracetam in healthy volunteer. *Ann Pharmacother* 2004;38(11):1816-22.

[124] Harden CL, Lazar LM, Pick LH, Nikolov B, Goldstein MA, Carson D, Ravdin LD, Kocsis JH, Labar DR.A beneficial effect on mood in partial epilepsy patients treated with gabapentin. *Epilepsia* 1999;40(8):1129-34.

[125] Meador KJ, Loring DW, Hulihan JF, Kamin M, Karim R, CAPSS-027 Study Group. Differential cognitive and behavioral effects of topiramate and valproate. *Neurology* 2003;40(9):1279-85.

[126] Roullet FI, Wollaston L, Decatanzaro D, Foster JA Behavioral and molecular changes in the mouse in response to prenatal exposure to the anti-epileptic drug valproic acid *Neuroscience* 2010;170(2):514-22.

[127] Xie X, Hagan RM.Cellular and molecular actions of lamotrigine: possible mechanisms of efficacy in bipolar disorder. *Neuropsychobiology* 1998;38(3):119-30.

[128] Trimble MR, Schmitz B. Forced Normalization and Alternative Psychoses of Epilepsy.Petersfield, UK: Wrightson Biomedical Publishing Ltd; 1998.

[129] Grivas A, Schramm J, Kral T, von Lehe M, Helmstaedter C, Elger CE, Clusmann H. Surgical treatment for refractory temporal lobe epilepsy in the elderly: seizure outcome and neuropsychological sequels compared with a younger cohort. *Epilepsia* 2006;47(8):1364-72.

[130] Gatzonis SD, Stamboulis E, Siafakas, Angelopoulos E, Georgaculias N, Sigounas E, Jekins A. Gatzonis SD, Stamboulis E, Siafakas, Angelopoulos E, Georgaculias N, Sigounas E, Jekins A. Acute psychosis and EEG normalisation after vagus nerve stimulation. *J Neurol Neurosurg Psychiatry* 2000;69(2):278-9.

[131] Olesen JB, Hansen PR, Erdal J, Abildstrøm SZ, Weeke P, Fosbøl EL, Poulsen HE, Gislason GH. Antiepileptic drugs and risk of suicide: a nationwide study. *Pharmacoepidemiol Drug Saf* 2010;19(5):518-24.

[132] Kalinin VV, Polyanskiy DA. Gender differences in risk factors of suicidal behavior in epilepsy *Epilepsy Behav* 2005;6(3):424-9.

[133] US Food and Drug Administration. Antiepileptic drugs and suicidality. 23-5-2008 [online]. Available from URL: http://www.fda.gov/ohrms/dockets/ac/08/ briefing/2008- 4372b1-01-FDA.pdf [Accessed 2008 Jun 30].

[134] Machado RA, Espinosa AG, Melendrez D, González YR, García VF, Rodríguez YQ. Suicidal risk and suicide attempts in people treated with antiepileptic drugs for epilepsy.*Seizure* 2011;20(4):280-4.

[135] Bradford HF.Glutamate, GABA and epilepsy. *Prog Neurobiol* 1995;47(6):477-511.

[136] Fakhoury TA, Miller JM, Hammer AE, Vuong A. Effects of lamotrigine on mood in older adults with epilepsy and co-morbid depressive symptoms: an open-label, multicentre, prospective study. *Drugs Aging* 2008;25(11):955-62.

[137] Cavanna AE, Ali F, Rickards HE, McCorry D. Behavioral and Cognitive Effects of Anti-epileptic Drugs. *Discovery medicine* 2010;9(45):138-44.

[138] Genton P, Van Vleymen B. Piracetam and levetiracetam: close structural similarities but different pharmacological and clinical profiles. *Epileptic Disord* 2000;2(2):99–105.

[139] Wolf P, Trimble MR. Biological antagonism and epileptic psychosis.*Br J Psychiatry* 1985;146:272-6.

[140] Wolf P. Acute behavioural symptomatology at disappearance of epileptiform EEG abnormality: paradoxical or forced normalization. In: Smith D, Treiman D, Trimble MR, eds. *Neurobehavioural problems in epilepsy*. New York: Raven Press, 1991.

[141] Boylan LS, Flint LA, Labovitz DL, Jackson SC, Starner K, Devinsky O. Depression but not seizure frequency predicts quality of life in treatment-resistant epilepsy. *Neurology.* 2004;62(2):258-61.

[142] Goldstein MA, Harden CL, Radvin LD. Does anxiety in epilepsy patients decrease with increasing seizure frequency?.*Epilepsia* 1999;40(Suppl8):60-1.

[143] Brodtkorb E, Mula M. Optimizing therapy of seizures in adult patients with psychiatric comorbidity. *Neurology* 2006;67(12 Suppl 4):S39-44.

[144] Puzynski S.Anticonvulsants (carbamazepine, valproate, lamotrigine) on bipolar affective disorder. *Psychiatr Pol* 2002;36(6 Suppl):53-61.

[145] Mishory A, Yaroslavsky Y, Bersudsky Y, Belmaker RH. Phenytoin as an antimanic anticonvulsant: a controlled study. *Am J Psychiatry* 2000;157(3):463-5.

[146] Dodrill CB, Arnett JL, Deaton R, Lenz GT, Sommerville KW. Tiagabine versus phenytoin and carbamazepine as add-on therapies: effects on abilities, adjustment, and mood. *Epilepsy Res 2000*;42(2-3):123-32.

[147] Blumer D. Antidepressant and double antidepressant treatment for the affective disorder of epilepsy. *J Clin Psychiatry* 1997;58(1):3–11.

[148] Ojemann LM, Friel PN, Trejo WJ, Dudley DL. Effect of doxepin on seizure frequency in depressed epileptic patients. *Neurology* 1982;33(5):646–8.

[149] Robertson MM, Trimble MR. The treatment of depression in patients with epilepsy. A double-blind trial. *J Affect Discord* 1985;9(2):127–36.

[150] Favale E, Rubino V, Mainardi P, Lunardi G, Albano C. Anticonvulsant effect of fluoxetine in humans. *Neurology* 1995;45(10):1926–27.

[151] Jabbari B, Bryan GE, Marsh EE, Gunderson CH. Incidence of seizures with tricyclic and tetracyclic antidepressants. *Arch Neurol* 1985;42(5):480–1.

[152] Jick SS, Jick H, Knauss TA, Dean AD. Antidepressants and convulsions. *J Clin Psychopharmacol* 1992;12(4):241–5.

[153] Hawton K, Bergen H, Simkin S, Cooper J, Waters K, Gunnell D, Kapur N. Toxicity of antidepressants: rates of suicide relative to prescribing and non-fatal overdose *Br J Psychiatry* 2010;196(5):354-8.

[154] Phillips S, Brent J, Kulig K, Heiligenstein, J., Birkett, M. Fluoxetine versus tricyclic antidepressants: a prospective multicenter study of antidepressant drug overdoses. The Antidepressant Study Group. *J Emerg Med* 1997;15(4):439–45.

[155] Harvey AT, Preskorn SH. Cytochrome P450 enzymes: interpretation of their interactions with selective serotonin reuptake inhibitors (part 1). *J Clin Psychopharmacol* 1996;16(4):273–85.

[156] Dursun SM, Mathew VM, Reveley MA. Toxic serotonin syndrome after fluoxetine plus carbamazepine. *Lancet* 1993;342(8868):442-3.

[157] McConnell H, Duncan D. Treatment of psychiatric comorbidity in epilepsy. In H McConnell, PJ Snyder (eds), Psychiatric Comorbidity in Epilepsy: *Basic Mechanisms, Diagnosis, and Treatment.* Washington, DC: American Psychiatric Press 1998:245–36.

[158] Rosenstein DL, Nelson JC, Jacobs SC. Seizures associated with antidepressants: a review. *J Clin Psychiatry* 1993;54(8):289–99.

[159] Grimsley SR, Jann MW, Carter JG, D'Mello AP, D'Souza MJ. Increased carbamazepine plasma concentrations after fluoxetine coadministration. *Clin Pharmacol Ther 1991*;50(1):10–5.

[160] Lucena MI, Blanco E, Corrales MA, Berthier ML. Interaction of fluoxetine and valproic acid. *Am J Psychiatry* 1998;155(4):575.

[161] Baghai TC, Möller HJ. Electroconvulsive therapy and its different indications. *Dialogues Clin Neurosci* 2008;10(1):105-17.

[162] Elger G, Hoppe C, Falkai P, Rush AJ, Elger CE. Vagus nerve stimulation is associated with mood improvements in epilepsy patients. *Epilepsy Res* 2000;42(2-3):203-10.

[163] Menza MA, Murray GB, Holmes VF, Rafuls WA. Controlled study of extrapyramidal reactions in the management of delirious, medically ill patients: intravenous haloperidol versus intravenous haloperidol plus benzodiazepines. *Heart Lung* 1988;17(3):238–41.

[164] Marder S. Antipsychotic medications. In AF Schatzberg, CB Nemeroff (eds), *Textbook of Psychopharmacology* (2nd ed). Washington, DC: American Psychiatric Press 1998;309–22.

[165] Marks RC, Luchins DJ. *Antipsychotic medications and seizures.* Psychiatr Med 1991;9(1):37–51.
[166] Denney D, Stevens JR. Clozapine and seizures. *Biol Psychiatry* 1995;37(7):425–6.
[167] Shukla S, Mukherjee S, Decina P. Lithium in the treatment of bipolar disorders associated with epilepsy: an open study. *J Clin Psychopharmacol* 1988;8(3):201–4.
[168] Ninan TN, Cole JO, Yonkers KA. Nonbenzodiazepine anxiolytics. In AF Schatzberg, CB Nemeroff (eds), *Textbook of Psychopharmacology* (2nd ed). Washington, DC: American Psychiatric Press 1998;287–300.
[169] Catalano G, Catalano MC, Hanley PF. Seizures associated with buspirone overdose: case report and literature review. *Clin Neuropharmacol* 1998;21(6):347–50.
[170] Yudofsky SC, Silver JM, Hales RE. Treatment of agitation and aggression. In SC Yudofsky, RE Hales (eds), *The American Psychiatric Press Textbook of Neuropsychiatry.* Washington, DC: American Psychiatric Press 1997:881–900.
[171] Raju SS, Gopalakrishna HN, Venkatadri N. Effect of propranolol and nifedipine on maximal electroshock-induced seizures in mice: individual and in combination. *Pharmacol Res* 1998;38(6):449–52.
[172] van der Feltz-Cornelis CM, Aldenkamp AP. Effectiveness and safety of methylphenidate in adult attention deficit hyperactivity disorder in patients with epilepsy: an open treatment trial. *Epilepsy Behav* 2006;8(3):659-62.
[173] Gross-Tsur V, Manor O, van der Meere J, Joseph A, Shalev RS. Epilepsy and attention deficit hyperactivity disorder: is methylphenidate safe and effective?. *J Pediatr* 1997;130(4):670-4.

In: Seizures and Anti-Epileptic Drugs
Editors: Willard Hosten and Aleph Burtsev

ISBN: 978-1-62100-255-0

Chapter II

Anti-Epileptic Drugs: Behavior and Cognition

Andrea E. Cavanna[1,2,*] *and Clare M. Eddy*[1]
[1]Department of Neuropsychiatry,
BSMHFT and University of Birmingham, UK
[2]Department of Neuropsychiatry,
Institute of Neurology and University College London, UK

Abstract

Anti-epileptic drugs (AEDs) are characterized by a variety of mechanisms of action, leading to different anticonvulsant activities and behavioral/psychotropic profiles. At the one end of the pharmacodynamic spectrum are AEDs potentiating inhibitory gamma-aminobutyric acid (GABA) neurotransmission. The other end of the spectrum comprises AEDs attenuating excitatory glutamate neurotransmission. GABA-enhancing AEDs have sedating and anti-manic effects, while the second group is characterized by antidepressant effects.

This chapter reviews the mechanisms of action, main clinical indications, and behavioral and cognitive profiles of a range of AEDs. In clinical practice, both patients' characteristics and AEDs' cognitive and behavioral profiles should be taken into account in order to maximize benefits in terms of seizure control and behavioral and cognitive outcome.

Keywords: Epilepsy, anticonvulsants, antiepileptic drugs, adverse effects, behavior, cognition

* Corresponding Author: Andrea Eugenio Cavanna, MD PhD. Department of Neuropsychiatry, University of Birmingham, Birmingham and Solihull Mental Health NHS Foundation Trust, Barberry Building, Birmingham B152FG, United Kingdom. Email: A.Cavanna@ion.ucl.ac.uk.

1. Introduction

Approximately two thirds of patients with epilepsy can achieve complete seizure freedom with the use of anti-epileptic drugs (AEDs), often after trialling a number of agents, sometimes in combination [1]. A range of different AEDs are currently available, which can be broadly categorised as older and newer agents.

Pharmacological Treatments for Epilepsy

Bromides were first used to treat seizures in the 1850s, and were followed by the common use of phenobarbital and phenytoin until the 1950s. Over the next couple of decades, sodium valproate and carbamazepine became popular treatments. These drugs, in addition to primidone and ethosuximide, were the six agents of choice until the 1990s, when a newer generation of drugs became available. There are now more than twenty different agents which are licensed for use in treating seizures in the UK.

Older AEDs have the advantages of lower cost, wide availability, and long-term experience. However, there are various drawbacks associated with these medications in terms of toxicity and adverse side effects. Some of the new AEDs differ from older agents in their mechanism of action, pharmacokinetic properties, efficacy spectrum, and adverse effects [2]. Side effects such as somnolence, nausea and dizziness are commonly experienced in association with the use of all AEDs. In general, newer agents are associated with better tolerance, but they can still exert a range of significant cognitive and behavioral effects.

Mechanisms of Action of Anti-epileptic Drugs

The psychotropic action of AEDs may be exerted via two distinct pathways. One pathway considers the mechanism of action of an AED to result from the interaction between the drug's effects and processes occurring in the brain in association with epilepsy. The other pathway involves the direct pharmacological effect of these drugs, broadly divided in two categories [3]. The more sedating AEDs typically augment gamma-aminobutyric acid (GABA) inhibitory transmission, resulting in effects such as cognitive slowing and drowsiness. Most older drugs (e.g. phenobarbital, valproate) are likely to form part of this category, in addition to newer agents, including gabapentin, tiagabine, vigabatrin and zonisamide. Other AEDs exert a more activating effect through the modulation of glutamate excitatory neurotransmission, and may possess potential positive effects on mood (e.g. lamotrigine, oxcarbazepine). Topiramate may have both kinds of effect.

Phenobarbital is a barbiturate (like its metabolite primidone) which binds to GABA receptors and potentiates the effect of GABA. Phenytoin is related to barbiturates and appears to block sodium channels limiting repetitive firing of action potentials. These actions can affect healthy neurons at toxic higher doses. Carbamazepine also stabilizes the inactivated state of sodium channels and can potentiate GABA receptors, and primidone is thought to work in a similar way. Sodium valproate may exert a slightly different action, by preventing the transamination of GABA (by inhibiting GABA transaminase) and blocking both voltage-gated sodium channels and T-type calcium channels. Ethosuximide is also thought to block calcium channels, although its exact mechanism of action is still unclear.

Tiagabine increases synaptic GABA by inhibiting its uptake into neurons and glia via inhibition of GAT-1GABA transporter, while vigabatrin is an irreversible inhibitor of GABA transaminase. Gabapentin is a cyclic GABA analogue. Its exact mechanism of action is unknown, but is likely to involve voltage-gated N-type calcium ion channels. The mechanism of action of pregabalin is thought to be similar to gabapentin, and involves reduction of neurotransmitter release through actions on proteins linked to voltage gated calcium channels. Clobazam is a benzodiazepine which enhances GABA-activated chloride currents at $GABA_A$-receptor-coupled Cl- channels.

Topiramate is a sulfamate-substituted monosaccharide. Actions that may contribute to its therapeutic effect include blockage of voltage-dependent sodium channels, augmentation of GABA activity at some GABA- A receptors, antagonism of AMPA/kainate subtype of the glutamate receptor, and inhibition of the carbonic anhydrase enzyme. Like topiramate, zonisamide, a sulphonamide derivative, possesses multiple mechanisms of action, including actions on T-type calcium channels and sodium channels.

The main anticonvulsant mechanism of action exerted by lamotrigine is thought to be prevention of excitatory neurotransmitter release through blocking voltage-dependent sodium channels. Oxcarbazepine may work in a similar way. Levetiracetam has a more novel mechanism of action and binds to synaptic vesicle protein 2A, which is believed to assist in synaptic vesicle exocytosis and neurotransmitter release. These actions ultimately inhibit glutamate transmission. Felbamate is another sodium channel blocker which inhibits glutamate neurotransmission. Unfortunately, potentially fatal aplastic anemia and hepatotoxicity have been linked to this agent [4], so it is rarely prescribed, restricting investigation of its cognitive and behavioral effects.

Factors Influencing Prescribing in Epilepsy

When prescribing AEDs to treat seizures, medication selection will depend on both patient profiles and specific drug characteristics.

Patients can present with a variety of seizure types. Seizures can be generalised (with the seizure discharge involving both hemispheres) or partial (with a focal discharge). Partial seizures can be simple (with no loss of consciousness) or complex (with loss of consciousness). Different seizure types can respond differently to particular agents. For example, phenytoin, carbamazepine and valproate can all be effective in treating generalised and partial seizures, although valproate may demonstrate reduced efficacy in ameliorating complex partial seizures [5]. Recommended AEDs for different seizure types are shown in Table 1.

Some of the most effective medications for seizures are associated with a considerable degree of toxicity. Vulnerabilities of the patients treated therefore need to be carefully considered. Differing metabolic profiles in children, the elderly or the acutely unwell may lead to caution [6]. The use of anticonvulsants during pregnancy is also of concern, in light of reported teratogenic effects such as cleft lip and cleft palate, and less frequently, subtle facial dysmorphism or "fetal anticonvulsant syndrome" [5].

Table 1. Currently recommended agents according to the National Institute for Health and Clinical Excellence Guidelines [149]

FOCAL ONSET EPILEPSY	
1st choice	Oxcarbazepine/carbazepine, lamotrigine, valproate, topiramate
2nd choice	Levetiracetam, phenytoin (acute situations), tiagabine, gabapentin, clobazam
GENERALIZED ONSET EPILEPSY	
1st choice	Valproate, ethosuximide (absence seizures), lamotrigine (low dose), carbamazepine (caution: myoclonus), topiramate
2nd choice	Levetiracetam, clobazam, oxcarbazepine

Further considerations include detrimental interactions with other medications the patient may be taking. For example, liver enzyme inducers (carbamazepine, phenytoin, phenobarbital, and primidone) compromise the efficacy of compounds metabolized along mutual pathways, including oral anti-coagulants, and antibacterials. The influence of AEDs on sex steroids and vitamin D metabolism also has the potential to lead to reproductive dysfunction and osteomalacia/osteoporosis. Most anticonvulsants induce the activity of hepatic enzymes, and this can result in the failure of contraceptive agents [5].

Effective treatment depends on medication compliance across a lifetime. Patient tolerability has been shown to be a significant limiting factor in the treatment of epilepsy, as adverse effects can lead to treatment withdrawal [7]. A drug's retention rate is therefore mainly determined by its side effect profile [1]. The adverse effects associated with AEDs range from transient and mild, to severe and potentially fatal complications. Although newer agents tend to be better tolerated, their use can still be limited by a number of negative behavioral and cognitive effects. A full appreciation of the behavioral and cognitive effects of AEDs is therefore essential in order to make informed treatment decisions.

In the remainder of this chapter, we review the scientific literature which has documented the effects of a range of AEDs on behavior and cognition. We summarise the available evidence with a view to guiding treatment practices. Finally, we consider the limitations of reviewed studies and highlight useful avenues for future research.

2. Cognitive Effects of Anti-epileptic Drugs

All major AEDs have been reported to be associated with adverse cognitive side effects [8] and the average rate of AED-related intolerable cognitive side effects (leading to dosage change or discontinuation) has been estimated at 12.8% [9]. The most commonly reported cognitive alterations are reduced attention, psychomotor slowing and impaired memory.

Older AEDs

Dose related impairment in attention and reaction time, performance IQ and short-term memory are frequently seen with phenobarbital [10]. Studies involving children with epilepsy have linked phenobarbital use to lower IQ [11,12], and discontinuation of the drug can improve total IQ (mainly affecting non-verbal items) [13]. Phenobarbital is considered to have worse cognitive effects than valproate or carbamazepine [14,15]. Compared to carbamazepine, primidone has been found to cause more adverse effects on motor performance and attention/concentration tests [16,17].

Phenytoin is implicated in dose-related declines in concentration, memory, visuomotor functions and mental speed [18]. Pulliainen and Jokelainen [19] found that phenytoin had negative effects on visually guided motor speed of both hands; moreover, individuals taking phenytoin did not perform as well as individuals taking carbamazepine on a visual memory task. However, these authors concluded that the long-term effects of phenytoin on cognition are relatively few and restricted mainly to some visually guided motor functions. Another study comparing phenytoin, carbamazepine and valproate in childhood epilepsy showed only minimal cognitive decrements were linked to phenytoin [20]. Two groups of 25 patients on carbamazepine or phenytoin monotherapy were compared in an open clinical investigation [21]. The results showed lower performance with phenytoin compared to carbamazepine on all tests measuring motor speed but not for tasks involving attention and memory.

The data for carbamazepine is rather mixed. Mild cognitive and psychomotor effects have been linked to carbamazepine [22], including deterioration in information processing speed, attention [23] and verbal fluency [24]. This AED has been associated with impaired memory in children [25].

Forsythe et al [20] reported that children treated with carbamazepine performed worse than children treated with valproate on memory tasks. However, another study [26] reported that the cognitive profiles of valproate and carbamazepine were similar, except for some aspects of attention and memory, for which individuals taking valproate scored better, and for some motor tests, for which individuals taking carbamazepine performed faster. Overall, these effects are mild as compared with phenytoin and phenobarbital.

A randomized, double-blind, placebo-controlled study [27] involving 150 epilepsy patients on AED monotherapy (mainly carbamazepine or valproate) found that drug discontinuation significantly improved performance on tests that required complex cognitive processing under time pressure, but not on more simple tasks of attention and reaction time. A later study, in which most patients were taking carbamazepine, reported similar findings [28]. Performance improved on verbal fluency, inhibition, language and reaction time tasks.

Valproate may have a more benign cognitive profile. One study reported no significant decline in neuropsychological performance after valproate, although a lack of practice effect on tasks could have indicated subtle changes in performance [29].

Another study reported no significant adverse or beneficial neuropsychological effects of valproate in 279 adults with epilepsy [30]. A review of the effects of sodium valproate on cognitive function concluded that this agent has minimal adverse cognitive effects [31], and any adverse cognitive effects are likely to be reversible [32]. However, a recent study by Glauser et al [33] reported that attentional dysfunction was more common with valproate than ethosuximide (in 49% of the children vs. 33%).

In another study [34] no side effects were observed in nine patients prescribed ethosuximide for partial epilepsy, and improvements in cognitive performance with the use of ethosuximide have been reported for individuals both with and without epilepsy [35,36]. With regards to cognition, ethosuximide may therefore prove a more favorable option than valproate.

Newer AEDs

Although various trials have demonstrated a low rate of adverse cognitive side effects of tiagabine, difficulties with concentration and language problems have been reported [37]. Another study [38] reported deterioration in verbal memory in association with tiagabine from three months after baseline tests. However, Dodrill et al [39] documented improved motor speed, concentration, and verbal fluency after tiagabine.

Vigabatrin has demonstrated few adverse cognitive effects when compared with placebo in double-blind, add-on studies of patients with epilepsy [40-42] and fewer adverse effects than carbamazepine in a small, open-label, randomized, parallel-group study [43]. Vigabatrin had no detrimental effects on cognitive functions at twelve months, and memory retrieval and mental flexibility improved significantly. In a double blind study involving 100 adult epilepsy patients, 52 taking vigabatrin and the rest placebo [44], there was a tendency for improvement on most tests of cognitive function: 15 showed improvement, 1 showed no change, and scores worsened for 5 tests. Overall, vigabatrin monotherapy seems well tolerated in relation to cognition [45]. However, its use is associated with asymptomatic visual field constriction [46], which affects 30-50% of patients [47].

Using tasks including digit span, mental arithmetic and reaction time, Patat et al [48] showed that clobazam had no detrimental effects on performance at 10mg doses, but could lead to moderate memory difficulties at a dosage of 30mg.

Another study reported no difference between performance of patients with epilepsy taking clobazam or carbamazepam on tests assessing intelligence, memory, attention, psychomotor speed and impulsivity [49].

Berent et al [50] reported difficulties with learning in association with zonisamide in a small, add-on study. Cognitive difficulties were also reported by an open-label investigation [51]. After one year of treatment, 16 patients (47%) reported cognitive deficits. Worse performance was apparent on tasks involving attention, memory and verbal fluency, and was related to dose. These authors concluded that zonisamide has adverse effects on cognition even after one year of treatment.

Martin et al [52] showed that gabapentin had no significant effects on attention, psychomotor speed, language or memory. Little or no cognitive impairment has also been reported by other studies [53, 54]. In a double-blind crossover study comparing gabapentin and carbamazepine [55], gabapentin produced fewer negative cognitive side effects than carbamazepine, and improved performance on many measures. However, a 12-week, randomized, double-blind study of these AEDs involving 23 healthy participants revealed effects on the digit-symbol and Stroop tests, and differences between carbamazepine and gabapentin were not significant [56].

In one study only 2 of 50 epilepsy patients taking pregabalin reported cognitive problems [57]. However, rather a different impression was given by a study involving 32 healthy individuals [58]. Pregabalin was associated with significant decrements in performance on three of six cognitive measures (digit-symbol test, Stroop, verbal fluency task). In another study of 24 healthy volunteers [59], pregabalin led to no significant effects on tests assessing reaction time and short term memory compared with placebo. A limited decrement was noted on arousal and divided attention tests, along with improvement relative to placebo in brake reaction time.

Cognitive side effects are relatively common in association with topiramate, which can lead to impaired concentration, psychomotor slowing, and specific language problems in both healthy and epilepsy populations [52,60-64]. In epilepsy patients, topiramate also has an effect on verbal and spatial working memory [65,66], word fluency, verbal processing and verbal IQ [67,68]. One open-label study [69] involving 53 children reported no effects on verbal memory or symbol-digit tests. However, another study [38] reported significant deterioration in verbal fluency, language comprehension, and working memory with topiramate. Martin et al [52] reported performance declines on tests of attention and word fluency in association with topiramate are greater in comparison to gabapentin and lamotrigine. 'Word-finding difficulties' can be experienced by around 10-33% of patients [52, 70].

In one study [71] topiramate use in a 50-year old woman with multiple seizure types was associated with executive difficulties, concentration problems, poor visuo-spatial short-term memory, ataxic dysarthria, word-finding difficulties and perseveration. Most difficulties with attention, inhibition, language, memory and visuo-spatial skills had remitted six weeks after cessation of treatment, and all at eight months. Other studies report improvements in cognitive measures after topiramate withdrawal [72]. One open study [73] reported that 18/37 patients (49%) experienced cognitive deficits such as impaired concentration, psychomotoric slowing, memory deficits, and dysphasia, with add-on topiramate. In four patients, they were reversible after dose reduction. However, some detrimental effects may persist. Rorsman and Kallen [74] report case studies of two patients. Topiramate was linked to impaired naming, auditory comprehension, visuospatial and working memory and problem solving in a 25 year-old woman with intractable partial seizures. After withdrawal, all except visuospatial memory and problem solving improved. The other patient, a 38 year-old man, showed difficulties including visuospatial memory and verbal learning, retention, and fluency with topiramate. After withdrawal, verbal learning was still impaired and the visuospatial deficit also had not completely reversed.

One study of healthy individuals showed topiramate can lead to selective, statistically significant declines on measures of attention and word fluency at acute doses [52]. This study found no performance changes with gabapentin and lamotrigine. The latter AED is largely well-tolerated and induces fewer adverse CNS effects as compared to older AEDs, although dose-related adverse effects include dizziness, sedation and diplopia.

One double-blind, placebo-controlled crossover study of 81 patients with refractory partial seizures demonstrated no adverse effect on cognition in association with lamotrigine [75] and other studies have reported similar findings [76]. A study involving 25 healthy adults showed lamotrigine to significantly better performance than carbamazepine on variables including memory, cognitive speed, and perception of cognitive performance [77]. Positive effects on cognitive function in epilepsy have also been reported [52, 78, 79]. Attention processes, short-term memory, and motor and mental speed were investigated in 25 epilepsy patients taking carbamazepine plus lamotrigine as add-on therapy [80]. There were no significant score decreases after adding lamotrigine, and most changes were in a positive direction.

Studies have indicated no deterioration in learning, memory, or attention in patients with epilepsy treated with oxcarbazepine [8, 82]. A randomized, double-blind, placebo-controlled, crossover study of healthy individuals treated with oxcarbazepine revealed slowed reaction times, but slightly improved cancellation task performance and feelings of improved attention and alertness [83]. There were no significant differences on neuropsychological measures during a double-blind, randomized, parallel design study of healthy volunteers comparing oxcarbazepine with phenytoin [84]. Another study reported no impairment of cognitive function after 4–12 months of oxcarbazepine [85].

In one study, the cognitive effects associated with levetiracetam in intractactable epilepsy were compared to topiramate [86]. There were no significant differences in cognition for these AEDs, and no significant negative effects were reported with the use of levetiracetam [87]. No significant changes in psychomotor function, memory, or information processing were found in a study of 10 patients when levetiracetam was added to carbamazepine or phenytoin [88]. However, levetiracetam seemed to improve reaction time, tapping rate and memory. A double-blind, randomized, crossover study of healthy adults reported significantly better performance across a neuropsychological battery for levetiracetam compared with carbamazepine [89].

Conclusion

The older agents likely to have the greatest cognitive toxic potential are phenobarbital and perhaps primidone. Carbamazepine has the potential to lead to mild but sometimes significant difficulties within a range of cognitive process including attention, psychomotor speed, language-related skills and memory, whilst cognitive effects associated with phenytoin are generally restricted to visually guided motor functions. Minimal difficulties are also likely with sodium valproate, and clobazam taken at low doses. Further investigation is needed, but ethosuximide may be the older drug which shows the best cognitive profile.

With regards to newer drugs, topiramate may have the most detrimental influence on cognition. Little data are available at present for zonisamide, but findings so far indicate that long term adverse effects are possible.

Study findings for tiagabine and pregabalin are relatively mixed, although executive difficulties noted in healthy individuals with pregabalin merit caution. Although there is only limited evidence that vigabatrin interferes with cognition and that it could have some beneficial effects, its use is restricted due to reported visual field defects. More favourable options include gabapentin and oxcarbazepine, which have been associated with only minor cognitive difficulties. Based on the evidence reviewed, the agents least likely to interfere with cognitive processes are levetiracetam and lamotrigine, of which the latter is associated with the best evidence of improved cognitive performance.

3. Behavioral Effects of Anti-Epileptic Drugs

AEDs may contribute to both positive and negative behavioral changes in epilepsy. 'Activating' effects such as alertness, agitation and hyperactivity may be most common in association with agents possessing glutamatergic effects, while 'deactivating' effects linked to drowsiness and apathy may result from a broad range of agents which alter GABA transmission.

Older AEDs

Phenobarbital is linked to exacerbation of symptoms of hyperactivity, irritability, lethargy and depression [10]. Laders et al [62] report that phenobarbital is associated with agitation, confusion, nervousness, hallucinations, insomnia and anxiety. Behavioral disorders associated with phenobarbital and primidone are common at low plasma levels [90]. In one study, children exhibited more hyperactivity when taking phenobarbital in comparison to valproic acid [14], and primidone has also been linked to hyperactivity in children [91]. Behavioral changes can include psychosis [92], and one case of catatonic schizophrenia was reported in association with primidone [93]. Compared to carbamazepine, primidone has been found more likely to cause depression [16] and can cause impotence and decreased libido [94].

Banu et al [95] investigated the use of phenobarbital and carbamazepine in 108 children with epilepsy. In 59 children there was no change in behavior, and in 16 behavior improved. Ten children experienced excessive restlessness and hyperactivity: 4 out of 54 in the phenobarbital group and 6 out of 54 in the carbamazepine group. Aggressive outbursts associated with carbamazepine were seen in one child, and irritability was linked to phenobarbital in another. However, behavior was improved overall. Pulliainen and Jokelainen [19, 96] reported that use of phenytoin and carbamazepine resulted in similar decreases in tension, depression, and bewilderment, while vigour increased. However, other reports indicate phenytoin can be associated with anxiety, aggression, fatigue, and depression [18].

Sodium valproate has been shown to alter affect and mood in 19% of treated patients [97] and can induce irritability and depressive symptoms [98]. Behavioral disturbances, including nervousness, irritability, depression, hallucinations, and psychosis may have idiosyncratic as well as dose-related components with the use of ethosuximide (35, 36].

Newer AEDs

Agitation and irritability have been reported with vigabatrin [99]. Hyperkinesia and agitation have been shown to occur most commonly in pediatric populations. In a study on the use of vigabatrin in childhood epilepsy, this agent led to side effects including drowsiness, restlessness and irritability in 13% of children [100]. Sheth et al [101] found that vigabatrin use led to severe aggressive agitation in three patients. A study reporting the effects of vigabatrin as add-on therapy in children and adolescents with severe refractory epilepsy reported behavioral side effects, including fatigue and apathy [102], while other similar studies have reported increased appetite [103].

Some estimates suggest behavioral side effects such as agitation, irritability, depression or psychosis are seen in 2-4% of cases [104], but depression may be more common in patients with past history of depression [99]. In one study of add-on vigabatrin [105] involving 73 patients with refractory epilepsies, treatment had to be discontinued by 6 months in 52% of the sample, and mood problems were the main reason for discontinuation in 12.3% of the total sample. Another study reported [44] psychiatric side effects were a common reason for withdrawal of vigabatrin. Agitation was reported by 14% and amnesia was experienced by 20% of adult patients, but more extreme adverse effects included confusion/delusions or psychosis in two patients, aggressive behavior in two patients and suicidal ideation in one.

Despite these behavioral difficulties, there was a tendency for improvement on most tests of cognitive function and mood.

Similar behavioral problems may be seen in children in association with gabapentin. Aggression and agitation have also been reported (although rarely) with gabapentin [106]. Lee et al [107], report that this agent can increase behavioral problems (e.g. aggression, defiance, hyperactivity) in children with baseline attention deficit-hyperactivity disorder (ADHD) or developmental delay. All behavioral changes were reversible. In a retrospective analysis of 90 patients with epilepsy taking gabapentin, just 1% reported depression, and 1% decreased libido [108]. Other clinical reports support the possibility of mood improvement (i.e. reduced anxiety or depression) as a result of gabapentin use [109]. Similarly, pregabalin can result in irritability and anxiety in a few patients, but may conversely improve anxiety symptoms in other individuals [57]. In a prospective, open-label study of pregabalin, add-on trial side effects were evident in 32% of the sample, with evidence of somnolence, and appetite and behavioral change [110].

In a study comparing tiagabine to placebo, this agent led to increased drowsiness, nervousness, difficulties in concentration and depression [111]. Other studies have reported aggression, irritability and lethargy [112], increased rates of depression [113] and even hallucinations and paranoia [114] in association with tiagabine. However, one study [39] reported evidence of favourable changes on assessments in the areas of adjustment and mood.

Clobazam can be linked to mood changes including aggression, irritability, depression and disinhibition [115]. Restlessness and undesirable destructive, antagonistic or impulsive behaviors have also been noted [116], which may be more prominent in children. In a 24-week open-labelled trial in adults with epilepsy [117], the commonest side effect was sedation, but weight gain, gait ataxia and loss of short-term memory were noted in a few patients. In children with intractable epilepsy [118], side effects were reported in 22.5%, including irritability and behavioral change.

A large retrospective study of 103 patients by Mula and Trimble [119] highlighted a variety of psychological and behavioral symptoms linked to topiramate, such as affective disorders, among which are depressed mood and euphoria, aggressivity, acute psychosis and agitation. Irritability, apathy and appetite changes may also be seen [1,120] and emotional lability has been reported by a number of studies [60, 61, 63]. Ballieux et al [71] report behavioral effects on a 50 year old woman with refractory epilepsy, including marked behavioral disinhibition and pronounced emotional instability. Topiramate often exerts ‘deactivating’ side effects [121]. One study [122] of 470 epilepsy patients who had taken topiramate showed that of adverse effects, cognitive and behavioral side effects were dominant, with mental slowing (27.6%), dysphasia (16.0%), and mood problems (agitation: 11.9%) most frequently reported. In another study [123], 170 adult epilepsy patients were started on adjunctive topiramate, which was discontinued in 51 (30%) patients. The most common side effects resulting in withdrawal included fatigue, irritability and depression.

Similar side effects have been reported in children. Mohamed et al [124] conducted a retrospective review of the use of topiramate in 51 children with epilepsy aged 3-16 years. Adverse effects were seen in 57% and led 20 to withdraw from treatment. The most common adverse effects included agitation/irritability (13%), depression (13%), lethargy (10%) and visual hallucinations (3%). A prospective clinical trial of topiramate [125] involving 47 children aged 6-60 months with refractory epilepsy reported mild to moderate adverse effects, mainly somnolence, anorexia and nervousness, in 53% of children.

Some studies have reported that only mild behavioral change and appetite loss are linked to zonisamide [126]. A prospective, randomized, open-label investigation of zonisamide monotherapy on cognition and mood in epilepsy [51] involved 43 patients with epilepsy but nine patients were withdrawn prior to follow-up. Three patients dropped out during the titration period because of cognitive and mood problems. However, overall only five patients (15%) experienced mood changes.

In another study [127] on 77 children with epilepsy treated with zonisamide, 39% reported side effects, including somnolence (11.7%), decreased spontaneity (7.8%) and anorexia (6.5%). Hirari et al [128] reported treating 27 children with epilepsy with zonisamide monotherapy over two years. Excellent seizure control was achieved, but two cases (7.4%) had behavior disturbances. The first was a 14-year-old girl with partial epilepsy who developed mutism, violent behavior and lack of concentration at 10 years of age. The second was a 15-year-old girl with generalized tonic-clonic seizures who developed obsessive compulsive disorders (OCD) when aged 13 years. Decreasing the dosage of zonisamide reduced these problems.

Several articles have noted significant behavioral side effects with zonisamide such as depression and psychotic episodes [129,130], although these have usually appeared during polytherapy. One review of zonisamide [131] found 14 of 74 patients had psychotic episodes. The risk was higher in young patients. In 13 patients, psychotic episodes occurred within a few years of commencement. In children, obsessive-compulsive symptoms appeared to be related to psychotic episodes.

A study involving 25 healthy adults found lamotrigine yielded significantly better performance on variables including mood factors and sedation in comparison to carbamazepine [77]. Although common side effects can include sedation, this drug appears to possess a 'mood activating' property, relative to both placebo and valproate [132]. Lamotrigine often improves alertness, irritability and emotional stability [1]. Mood improvements have been reported in numerous open clinical studies [75, 133, 134] and lamotrigine has been documented as having broad-spectrum efficacy in depression, hypomania and mixed phases of bipolar disorder [135]. Evidence from clinical studies further indicates the efficacy of lamotrigine in alleviating affective symptoms in patients with epilepsy [136].

In one quarter of a sample of 83 children with focal or generalized epilepsy, lamotrigine was associated with increased alertness and improved behavior regardless of seizure control [137]. Side effects were relatively uncommon. In the previously cited study by Bootsma et al [120], behavioral side effects were reported by a limited number of patients who chose to discontinue treatment. These included agitation (3.4%), aggression (2.4%), irritability (2.5%), confusion (0.8%), depression (0.4%) and apathy (0.4%). Overall, lamotrigine is associated with little evidence of adverse cognitive or behavioral effects [62].

Oxacarbazepine is occasionally linked to side effects such as fatigue and drowsiness [138, 139] but few cognitive or behavioral effects have been reported. Franzoni et al [140] reported agitation in one patient and memory difficulties in another. However, mood improvement similar to that generated by lamotrigine has been reported in children treated with oxcarbazepine [141].

Behavioral symptoms linked to levetiracetam include agitation, anti-social behavior, anxiety, apathy, depersonalization, depression, emotional lability, euphoria, hostility, nervousness, neurosis, and personality disorder [142]. Data from 1,023 patients with epilepsy treated with levetiracetam [143] showed increased affective symptoms in the domains of anxiety, hostility, emotional lability, depression and nervousness. A retrospective study of add-on treatment in 80 patients with focal epilepsy reported that somnolence and aggressiveness were common side effects [144]. Similar findings were reported in children with epilepsy in an add-on open label trial [145]. Mild to moderate side effects were reported in 128 patients (44.9%), consisting most frequently of somnolence (23.9%), general behavioral changes (15.4%), aggression (10.5%) and sleep disturbance (3.2%). Neurologically handicapped children showed an increased risk for reversible neurocognitive side effects.

Bootsma et al [122] report that the most prevalent adverse effects associated with levetiracetam are agitation, aggression, irritability and tiredness. Some patients can also experience improved mood, such as feeling cheerful, calm or active, while others may report depression or apathy. In one study [146] 7% of patients reported positive behavioral effects such as feeling more energetic, active and cheerful. 'Activating' mood-changes were reported by 13.8% and 'de-activating' effects by 13.1%. Adverse behavioral effects were more common in cases with mental handicap.

Studies of children have also highlighted possible beneficial behavioral effects. In an open, retrospective study involving 133 children with refractory epilepsy [7], side effects were seen in 27.8% of cases, but were usually transient or tolerable. In 37 children, relatives noted improvement in their social behavior and cognitive abilities. Similar findings were reported by another retrospective open trial of levetiracetam [147] involving 43 children and adolescents with refractory epilepsies. Relatives noted an improvement in social behavior and in cognitive skills in the case of 15 children (34.9%). Another study reported that while levetiracetam (as add-on or monotherapy) was linked to tiredness (in 7.8% of children with epilepsy) and aggressiveness (in 5%), a positive effect on behavior and/or alertness was apparent in 25% of patients [148].

Conclusion

Older agents such as phenobarbital and primidone can often lead to hyperactivity in children, and have also been linked to psychosis. The negative behavioral effects linked to carbamazepine appear less frequent and milder, while mixed evidence suggests phenytoin can have both positive and negative behavioral effects. A range of difficulties have been linked to clobazam, although children may be more susceptible. Limited data are available in relation to valproate and ethosuximide, so it is difficult to fully evaluate these agents. However, the data which are available already indicate the potential for at least some adverse effects including irritability and depression, beyond the well known antimanic effects of valproate.

Of the newer agents, available data indicate topiramate could have the widest variety of adverse behavioral effects, which include agitation, aggression, depression, emotional lability, disinhibition and psychosis. These effects may be more likely to lead to withdrawal than milder effects associated with other agents. Psychosis has also been linked to zonisamide, although studies investigating this AED have provided somewhat mixed results, and in some cases behavioral side effects appear mild. Difficulties may be more common in children, in whom zonisamide can be linked to appetite changes, obsessive compulsive symptoms and decreased spontaneity.

While tiagabine has been linked to side effects including irritability, aggression, depression and psychosis, the data are mixed, because mood improvements have also been reported. Studies report similar findings for vigabatrin, as agitation and irritability or aggression have been reported in children and mood changes (including depression) can be seen in adults, although some positive effects have also been reported. Clobazam may exert problematic effects in children more often than adults, including restlessness, disinhibition and impulsive behavior. However, reports indicate these difficulties do not generally warrant discontinuation.

Fewer difficulties are associated with gabapentin and pregabalin. It has been suggested that behavioral difficulties may be more likely with gabapentin in children who already exhibit behavioural problems, and that this drug could help with anxiety or depression in adults. Pregabalin is associated with mild irritability in a few patients but could also assist with anxiety.

Levetiracetam has also been linked to a wide variety of behavioral effects such as personality changes, apathy, and depersonalisation, which are rarely seen with other AEDs. Aggression may be a more common side effect, although children with existing behavioral difficulties may be most susceptible. Conversely, some positive effects have been noted in children, including increased alertness and more sociable behavior. In general, lamotrigine appears to have positive effects on alertness, mood and emotional stability, and has been linked to negative behavioral effects in only a small minority of patients. Oxcarbazepine is another AED which appears to have minimal adverse effects and potential therapeutic influences on mood and behavior.

Conclusion

Summary of Study Findings

All AEDs have the potential to exert adverse cognitive and behavioral effects. In general, the sedating effects of AEDs with GABAergic mechanisms may interfere more with cognition, with older agents exerting more detrimental effects than newer drugs. In relation to behavioral side effects, positive effects including potential anxiolytic and antidepressant properties may be most likely in association with newer agents which attenuate glutamate excitatory neurotransmission. Having said this, the data reviewed suggest an AED's identified mode of action may not always predict its cognitive or behavioral profile. This could partly reflect the fact that the mechanisms of action of many AEDs are not yet fully understood, and observed effects could be exerted by unknown mechanisms of action.

Importantly, the data reviewed indicate that the behavioral effects exerted by an AED are likely to vary depending on factors linked to patient characteristics and individual susceptibility. Cognitive and behavioral problems already present can be exacerbated by some AEDs. For example, depressive effects may be more common in those individuals with a history of depression, and neurocognitive effects may be more common in individuals with existing learning difficulties.

This review has also shown that differing behavioral presentations may result from the same neuropharmacological effects in children and adults, and AEDs could have the potential to exert differing cognitive and behavioral effects across the lifespan. Hyperactivity effects appear more common in children than adults, who may simply experience increased alertness, and mood effects such as depression may be more easily recognised in adults than children. The cognitive influence of AEDs could be of greater significance to younger individuals, given that some of these agents may have the potential to interfere with learning and cognitive development.

Limitations and Recommendations for Future Research

The data reviewed suggest that agents such as phenobarbital and topiramate may have most detrimental impact on cognition and behavior in epilepsy. However, it is difficult to compare findings across studies due to variation in study design, treatment group and assessment tools. Analysis is also limited by the availability of studies for particular agents. Many investigations have been conducted into agents including topiramate, while there are limited data available for AEDs such as ethosuximide and oxcarbazepine.

Many studies are conducted with groups of patients exhibiting refractory epilepsy, who may constitute a severe subgroup of patients not representative of the entire population [6]. Where studies have assessed the use of the drugs in particular populations such as healthy adults, children with epilepsy, learning disabilities, different seizure types, epilepsy after brain injury etc., the side effects reported by these studies will at least partly reflect the differing clinical characteristics and specific vulnerabilities of these groups.

In relation to the current review, it is perhaps more difficult to draw conclusions from behavioral data. Indeed, it is more difficult to differentiate between the agents discussed based on these findings. In some cases there could be age differences in effects, which could partly reflect the assessment of children through behavioral observation and parent report in comparison to adult patients' self report. It is also difficult to determine whether reported changes in mood are linked to drug efficacy in treating seizures rather that direct effects on mood *per se*.

A number of randomized double-blind trials have been conducted. These studies appear favorable as they control for bias, although this approach could lack ecological validity. Add-on trials may be most problematic because of a possible increase the incidence of side effects due to potentiation of toxicity.

Longer term investigations are useful, because individuals may gradually develop tolerance to an AED's side effects. It is also informative for studies to investigate whether performance alters on discontinuation in order to determine if effects are reversible. Systematic trials are needed which compare the effects of commonly prescribed agents across subgroups of patients with epilepsy. Furthermore, little is known about the effects of AEDs in patients with seizures which cause specific alterations of the ictal conscious state [150]. Those studies involving children and adolescents of a wide range of ages should consider the potential impact of developmental change. Comparing age defined subgroups could also be useful as drug effects are likely to differ between younger and older children.

Based on the available evidence, a wide range of assessments clearly need to be included in future research. Studies investigating cognition should include tests of a range of executive functions including working memory, verbal fluency, inhibition, set-shifting and measures assessing transient, sustained and divided attention, short and long term aspects of verbal and visual memory, and motor functioning including dexterity and reaction time tests. Behavioral and psychiatric effects are also varied, and the investigation of these merit the inclusion of instruments to assess euthymic and dysthymic mood, agitation, irritability, aggressiveness, impulsivity, anxiety, sleep, appetite and signs of psychosis. Scales measuring hyperactive symptoms and obsessive compulsive behavior may also be of use for children. These scales should be age appropriate, and experimenters should consider the source of information, using both self and proxy rated instruments where possible. Further advancement in our understanding of the cognitive and behavioral impact of AEDs will be achieved through the development of specific instruments which are sensitive to the range of neuropsyhological and psychiatric effects exerted by these agents.

References

[1] Bootsma, HP; Rocker, L; Hekster, YA; Hulsman, J; Lambrechts, D; Majoie, M; Schellekens, A; de Krom, M; Aldenkamp, AP. The impact of side effects on long term retention in three new antiepileptic drugs. *Seizure,* 18, 327-331.

[2] Bourgeois, BFD. Anti-epileptic drugs, learning and behaviour in childhood epilepsy. *Epilepsia*, 1998, 39(9), 913-921.

[3] Ketter, TA; Post, RM; Theodore, WH. Positive and negative effects of antiepileptic drugs in patients with seizure disorders. *Neurology,* 1999, 53(5:S2), S53-S76.

[4] Bialer, M; Johannessen, SI; Kupferberg, HJ; Levy, RH; Perucca, E; Tomson, T. Progress report on new anti-epileptic drugs: a summary of the Eight Eilat Conference (EILAT-VIII). *Epilepsy Research,* 2007, 73, 1-52.

[5] Ropper, AH; Brown, RH. *Adams and Victor's Principles of Neurology*, 8th edition. London: McGraw Hill, 2005.

[6] Anderson, J; Moor, C-C. Anti-epileptic drugs: a guide for the non-neurologist. Clinical Medicine, 2010, 10(1), 24-58.

[7] Chung, S; Wang, N; Hank, N. Comparative retention rates and long-term tolerability of new antiepileptic drugs. *Seizure,* 2007, 16, 296-304.

[8] Aldenkamp, AP. Effects of antiepileptic drugs on cognition. *Epilepsia* 2001, 42(S1), 46-49.

[9] Arif, H; Buchsbaum, R; Weintraub, D; Pierro, J; Resor, SR; Hirsch, LJ. Patient-reported cognitive side effects of antiepileptic drugs: Predictors and comparison of all commonly used antiepileptic drugs. *Epilepsy and Behavior* 2009, 14(1), 202-209.

[10] Kwan, P; Brodie, MJ. Neuropsychological effects of epilepsy and antiepileptic drugs. *The Lancet,* 2001, 357, 216-222.

[11] Farwell, JR; Lee, YJ; Hirtz, DG; Sulzbacher, SI; Ellenberg, JH; Nelson, KB. Phenobarbital for febrile seizures-effects on intelligence and on seizure recurrence. *New England Journal of Medicine,* 1990, 322, 364-369.

[12] Camfield, CS; Chaplin, S; Doyle, AB; Shapiro, SH; Cummings, C; Camfield, PR. Side effects of phenobarbital in toddlers; behavioural and cognitive aspects. *Journal of Pediatrics,* 1979, 95, 361-365.

[13] Tonekaboni, SH; Beyraghi, N; Tahbaz, HS; Bahreynian, SA; Ashamohammadpoor, M. Neurocognitive effects of phenobarbital discontinuation in epileptic children. *Epilepsy and Behavior,* 2006, 8(1), 145-148.

[14] Vining, EPG; Mellits, ED; Dorsen, MM; Cataldo, MF; Quaskey, SA; Spielberg, SP; Freeman, JM. Psychologic and behavioural effects of antiepileptic drugs in children: a double-blind comparison between phenobarbital and valproic acid. *Pediatrics,* 1987, 80, 165-174.

[15] Calandre, EP; Dominguez-Granados, R; Gomez-Rubio, M; Molina-Font, JA. Cognitive effects of long-term treatment with Phenobarbital and valproic acid in school children. *Acta Neurologica Scandinavica* 1990, 81, 504-506.

[16] Rodin, EA; Rim, CS; Kitano, H; Lewis, R; Rennick, PM. A comparison of the effectiveness of primidone versus carbamazepine in epileptic outpatients. *The Journal of Nervous and Mental Disease,* 1976, 163(1), 41-46.

[17] Smith, DB; Mattson, RH; Cramer, JA; Collins, JF; Novelly, RA; Craft, B. Results of a nationwide Veterans Administration Cooperative Study comparing the efficacy and toxicity of carbamazepine, phenobarbital, phenytoin, and primidone. *Epilepsia,* 1987, 28, S50-S58.

[18] Gillham, RA; Williams, N; Wiedmann, KD; Butler, E; Larkin, JG; Brodie, MJ. Cognitive function in adult epileptic patients established on anticonvulsant monotherapy. *Epilepsy Research,* 1990, 7(3), 219-225.

[19] Pulliainen, V; Jokelainen, M. Comparing the Cognitive Effects of Phenytoin and Carbamazepine in Long-Term Monotherapy: A Two-Year Follow-Up. *Epilepsia,* 1995, 36(12), 1195-1202.

[20] Forsythe, I; Butler, R; Berg, I; McGuire, R. Cognitive impairment in new cases of epilepsy randomly assigned to carbamazepine, phenytoin and sodium valproate. *Developmental Medicine and Child Neurology,* 1991, 33, 524-34.

[21] Aldenkamp, AP; Alpherts, WCJ; Diepman, L; Vantslot, B; Overweg, J; Vermeulen, J. Cognitive side-effects of phenytoin compared with carbamazepine in patients with localization related epilepsy. *Epilepsy Research,* 1994, 19(1), 37-43.

[22] Gillham, RA; Williams, N; Wiedmann, KD; Butler, E; Larkin, JG; Brodie, MJ. Concentration-effect relationships with carbamazepine and its epoxide on psychomotor and cognitive function in epileptic patients. *Journal of Neurology, Neurosurgery and Psychiatry,* 1988, 51, 929-933.

[23] Wesnes, KA; Edgar, C; Dean, ADP; Wroe, SJ. The cognitive and psychomotor effects of remacemide and carbamazepine in newly diagnosed epilepsy. *Epilepsy and Behaviour,* 2009, 14(3), 522-528.

[24] Aikiä, M; Jutila, L; Salmenperä, T; Mervaala, E; Kälviäinen, R. Comparison of the cognitive effects of tiagabine and carbamazepine as monotherapy in newly diagnosed adult patients with partial epilepsy: pooled analysis of two long-term, randomized, follow-up studies. *Epilepsia,* 2006, 47(7), 1121-1127.

[25] Seidel, WT; Mitchell, WG. Cognitive and Behavioral Effects of Carbamazepine in Children: Data from Benign Rolandic Epilepsy. *Journal of Child Neurology,* 1999, 14(11), 716-723.

[26] Coenen, AML; Konings, GMLG; Aldenkamp, AP; Reiner, WO; van Luijtelaar, ELJM. Effects of chronic use of carbamazepine and valproate on cognitive processes. *Journal of Epilepsy,* 1995, 8(3), 250-254.

[27] Hessen, E; Lossius, MI; Reinvang, I; Gjerstad, L. Influence of Major Antiepileptic Drugs on Attention, Reaction Time, and Speed of Information Processing: Results from a Randomized, Double-blind, Placebo-controlled Withdrawal Study of Seizure-free Epilepsy Patients Receiving Monotherapy. *Epilepsia,* 2006, 47(12), 2038-2045.

[28] Hessen, E; Lossius, MI; Gjerstad, L. Antiepileptic monotherapy significantly impairs normative scores on common tests of executive functions. *Acta Neurologica Scandinavica* 2009, 119, 194-198.

[29] Prevey, ML; Delaney, RC; Cramer, JA; Cattanach, L; Collins, JF; Mattson, RH. Effect of valproate on cognitive functioning: comparison with carbamzepine. *Archives of Neurology,* 1996, 53(10), 1008-1016.

[30] Dikmen, SS; Machamer, JE; Winn, HR; Anderson, GD; Temkin, NR. Neuropsychological effects of valproate in traumatic brain injury: a randomized trial. *Neurology,* 2000, 54(4), 895-902.

[31] Trimble, MR; Thompson, PJ. Sodium valproate and cognitive function. *Epilepsia,* 1984, 25(S1), S60-S64.

[32] Galassi, R; Morreale, A; Lorusso, S; Procaccianti, G; Lugaresi, E; Baruzzi, A. Cognitive effects of valproate. *Epilepsy Research,* 1990, 5(2), 160-164.

[33] Glauser, TA; Cnaan, A; Shinnar, S; Hirtz, DG; Dlugos, D; Masur, D; Clark, PO; Capparelli, EV; Adamson, PC. (for the Childhood Absence Epilepsy Study Group). Ethosuximide, Valproic Acid, and Lamotrigine in Childhood Absence Epilepsy. *New England Journal of Medicine* 2010, 362, 790-799.

[34] Capovilla, G; Beccaria, F; Veggiotti, P; Rubboli, G; Meletti, S; Tassinari, CA. Ethosuximide is effective in the treatment of epileptic negative myoclonus in childhood partial epilepsy. *Journal of Child Neurology,* 1999, 14(6), 395-400.

[35] Browne, TR; Dreifuss, FE; Dyken, PR; Goode, DJ; Penry, JK; Porter, RJ; White, BG; White, PT. Ethosuximide in the treatment of absence (petit mal) seizures. *Neurology* 1975, 25, 515–524.

[36] Glauser, TA. Succinimides: Adverse Effects. In: Levy, RH; Mattson, RH; Meldrum, BS (Eds.). *Antiepileptic Drugs* (pp. 658–664). 5th edition. Philadelphia: Lippincott, Williams and Wilkins, 2002.

[37] Kalviainen, R. Long-term safety of tiagabine. *Epilepsia,* 2001, 42(S3), 46-48.

[38] Fritz, N; Glogau, S; Hoffmann, J; Rademacher, M; Elger, CE; Helmstaedter, C. Efficacy and cognitive side effects of tiagabine and topiramate in patients with epilepsy. *Epilepsy and Behavior,* 2005, 6(3), 373-381.

[39] Dodrill, CB; Arnett, JL; Shu, V; Pixton, GC; Lenz, GT; Sommerville, KW. Effects of tiagabine on abilities, adjustment and mood. *Epilepsia,* 1998, 39(1), 33-42.

[40] Dodrill, CB; Arnett, JL; Sommerville, KW; Sussman, NM. Evaluation of the effects of vigabatrin on cognitive abilities and quality of life in epilepsy. *Neurology,* 1993, 43, 2501-2507.

[41] Dodrill, CB; Arnett, JL; Sommerville, KW; Sussman, NM. Effects of differing dosages of vigabatrin (SABRIL) on cognitive abilities and quality of life in epilepsy. *Epilepsia,* 1995, 36, 164-173.

[42] Gillham, RA; Blacklaw, J; McKee, PJW; Brodie, MJ. Effect of vigabatrin on sedation and cognitive function in patients with refractory epilepsy. Journal of Neurology, *Neurosurgery and Psychiatry*, 1993, 56, 1271-1275.

[43] Kalviainen, R; Aikia, M; Saukkonen, AM; Mervaala, E; Riekkinen, PJ. Vigabatrin versus carbamazepine monotherapy in patients with newly diagnosed epilepsy: a randomized controlled study. *Archives of Neurology,* 1995, 52, 989-996.

[44] Guberman, A; Bruni, J. Long-term open multicentre, add-on trial of vigabatrin in adult resistant partial epilepsy. *Seizure*, 2000, 9, 112-118.

[45] Ylinen, A; Kalviainen, R; Riekkinen, PJ. Long term efficacy and cognitive effects of vigabatrin. *Acta Neurologica Scandinavica,* 1995, 92(S162), 47-50.

[46] Hemming, K; Maguire, MJ; Hutton, JL; Marson, AG. Vigabatrin for refractory partial epilepsy. *Cohrane Database of Systematic Reviews,* 2008, 3, CD007302.

[47] Gonzalez, PA; McCall, A; McQuistan, A; Keating, D; Brodie, MJ; Parks, S. Assessing retinal toxicity of vigabatrin and other gaba-ergic drugs in patients with epilepsy. *Association for Research in Vision and Ophthalmology,* 2006, 1658, B521.

[48] Patat, A; Klein, MJ; Surjus, A; Rostand, A; Granier, J. Study of effects of clobazam and lorazepam on memory and cognitive functions in healthy subjects. *Human Psychopharmacology: Clinical and Experimental,* 1991, 6(3), 229-241.

[49] Bawden HN and the Canadian Study Group for childhood Epilepsy. The cognitive and behavioural effects of clobazam and standard monotherapy are comparable. Epilepsy Re*search*, 1999, 33(2-3), 133-43.

[50] Berent, S; Sackellares, JC; Giordani, B; Wagner, JC; Donofrido, PD; Abuo-Khalil, B. Zonisamide (CI-912) and cognition: results from preliminary study. *Epilepsia*, 1987, 28, 61-67.

[51] Park, SP; Hwang, YH; Lee, HW; Suh, CK; Kwon, SH; Lee, BI. Long-term cognitive and mood effects of zonisamide monotherapy in epilepsy patients. *Epilepsy and Behavior,* 12(1), 102-108.

[52] Martin, R; Kuzniecky, R; Ho, S; Hetherington, H; Pan, J; Sinclair, K; Gilliam, F; Faught, E. Cognitive effects of topiramate, gabapentin, and lamotrigine in healthy young adults. *Neurology* 1999, 52, 321-7.

[53] Leach, JP; Girvan, J; Paul, A; Brodie, MJ. Gabapentin and cognition: a double blind, dose ranging, placebo controlled study in refractory epilepsy. *Journal of Neurology, Neurosurgery and Psychiatry,* 1997, 62(4), 372-376.

[54] Meador, KJ; Loring, DW; Ray, PG; Murrow, AM; King, DW; Nichols, ME; Deer, EM; Goff, WT. Differential cognitive effects of carbamazepine and gabapentin. *Epilepsia,* 1999, 40, 9, 1279-1285.

[55] Meador, KJ. Cognitive effects of epilepsy and of antiepileptic medications. In: *The Treatment of Epilepsy.* Wyllie, E (Ed.). Baltimore: Williams and Wilkins; 2005.

[56] Salinsky, MC; Binder, LM; Oken, BS; Storzbach, D; Aron, CR; Dodrill, CB. Effects of gabapentin and carbamazepine on the EEG and cognition in healthy volunteers. *Epilepsia,* 2002, 43(5), 482-490.

[57] Valentin, A; Moran, N; Hadden, R; Oakes, A; Elwes, R; Delamont, R; Mullatti, N; Naschef, L. Pregabalin as adjunctive therapy for partial epilepsy: An audit study in 96 patients from the South East of England. *Seizure,* 2009, 18, 450-452.

[58] Salinsky, M; Storzbach, D; Munoz, S. Cognitive effects of pregabalin in healthy volunteers: a double-blind, placebo-controlled trial. *Neurology, 2010*, 74(9), 755-61.

[59] Hindmarch, I; Trick, L; Ridout, F. A double-blind, placebo- and positive-internal-controlled (alprazolam) investigation of the cognitive and psychomotor profile of pregabalin in healthy volunteers. *Psychopharmacology,* 2005, 183(2), 133-143.

[60] Burton, LA. Effect of topiramate on attention. *Epilepsy Research,* 1997, 27(1), 29-32.
[61] Glauser, TA. Topiramate. *Epilepsia,* 1999, 40(S5), S71-S80.
[62] Laders, CM; Schraeder, PL; Claycamp, HG. Clinical Pharmacology of Topiramate versus Lamotrigine versus Phenobarbital: Comparison of Efficacy and Side Effects Using Odds Ratios. *Journal of Clinical Pharmacology*, 2003, 43, 491.
[63] Mula, M; Cavanna, AE; Trimble, M. Psychopharmacology of topiramate: from epilepsy to bipolar disorder. *Neuropsychiatric Disease and Treatment,* 2006, 2(4), 475-488.
[64] Perucca, E. A pharmacological and clinical review on topiramate, a new antiepileptic drug. *Pharmacological Research,* 1997, 35(4), 241-256.
[65] Jung, J-Y; Cho, J-W; Joo, EY; Kim, SH; Choi, KM; Chin, J; Park, K-W; Hong, SB. Cognitive effects of topiramate revealed by standardised low-resolution brain electromagnetic tomography (sLORETA) of event-related potentials. *Clinical Neurophysiology,* 2010, 1494-1501.
[66] Roy, C; Schwarzman, LK; Hulihan, JF; Xiang, J; Rosenthal, NR. Adjunctive topiramate therapy in patients receiving a mood stabilizer for bipolar I disorder: a randomized, placebo-controlled trial. *The Journal of Clinical Psychiatry*, 2006, 67(11), 1698–1706.
[67] Lee, S; Sziklas, V; Andermann, F; Farnham, S; Risee, G; Gustafson, M; Gates, J; Penovich, P, Al-Asmi, A; Dubeau, F; Jones-Gotman, M. The effects of adjunctive topiramate on cognitive function in patients with epilepsy. *Epilepsia,* 2003, 44, 339–347.
[68] Thompson, PJ; Baxendale, SA; Duncan, JS; Sander, JWAS. Effects of topiramate on cognitive function. *Journal of Neurology, Neurosurgery and Psychiatry,* 2000, 69, 636-641.
[69] Brandl, U; Kurlemann, G; Neubauer, B; Rettig, K; Schauble, B; Schreiner, A. Seizure and Cognitive Outcomes in Children and Adolescents with Epilepsy Treated with Topiramate. *Neuropediatrics,* 2010, 41(3), 113-120.
[70] Shorvon, SD. Safety of topiramate: adverse events and relationships to dosing. *Epilepsia,* 1996, 37(S2), 18-22.
[71] Baillieux, H; Verslegers, W; Paquier, P; De Deyn, PP; Marien, P. Cerebellar cognitive affective syndrome associated with topiramate. *Clinical Neurology and Neurosurgery,* 2008, 110, 496-499.
[72] Kockelmann, E; Elger, CE; Helmstaedter, C. Significant improvement in frontal lobe associated neuropsychological functions after withdrawal of topiramate in epilepsy patients. *Epilepsy Research,* 2003, 54, 171–178.
[73] Huppert, HJ; Quiske, A; Schulze-Bonhage, A. Cognitive impairment in add-on therapy with topiramate. *Nervenartz,* 2001, 72(4), 275.
[74] Rorsman, I; Kallen, K. Recovery of cognitive and emotional functioning following withdrawl of topiramate maintenance therapy. *Seizure,* 2001, 10, 592-595.
[75] Smith, D; Baker, G; Davies, G; Dewey, M; Chadwick, DW. Outcomes of add-on treatment with lamotrigine in partial epilepsy. *Epilepsia*, 1993, 34, 312-22.
[76] Gillham, R; Kane, K; Bryant-Comstock, L; Brodie, MJ. A double blind comparison on lamotrigine and carbamazepine in newly diagnosed epilepsy with quality of life as an outcome measure. *Seizure,* 2000, 9, 375-379.
[77] Meador, K; Loring, DW; Ray, PG; Murrow, AM; King, DW; Perrine, KR; Vazquez, BR; Kiolbasa, T. Differential cognitive and behavioural effects of carbamazepine and lamotrigine. *Neurology* 2001, 56, 1177–1182.

[78] Banks, GK; Beran, RG. Neuropsychological assessment in lamotrigine treated epileptic patients. *Clinical and Experimental Neurology,* 1991, 28, 230-237.

[79] Placidi, F; Marciani, MG; Diomedi, M; et al. Effects of lamotrigine on nocturnal sleep, daytime somnolence and cognitive functions in focal epilepsy. *Acta Neurologica Scandinavica* 2000, 102, 81-86.

[80] Aldenkamp, AP; Mulder, OG; Overweg, J. Cognitive effects of lamotrigine as first-line add-on in patients with localization-related (partial) epilepsy. *Journal of Epilepsy,* 1997, 10(3), 117-121.

[81] McKee, PJ; Blacklaw, J; Forrest, G; Gillham, RA; Walker, SM; Connelly, D; Brodie, MJ . A double-blind, placebo-controlled interaction study between oxcarbazepine and carbamazepine, sodium valproate and phenytoin in epileptic patients. British *Journal of Clinical Pharmacology,* 1994, 37, 27-32.

[82] Sabers, A; Moller, A; Dam, M; Smed, A; Arlien-Soborg, P; Buchman, J; Anderson, EB; Boesen, F; Dam, AM; Lyon, BB et al. Cognitive function and anticonvulsant therapy: effect of monotherapy in epilepsy. *Acta Neurologica Scandinavica,* 1995, 92, 19-27.

[83] Curran, HV; Java R. Memory and psychomotor effects of oxcarbazepine in healthy human volunteers. *European Journal of Clinical Pharmacology,* 1993, 44, 529-533.

[84] Salinsky, MC; Spencer, DC; Oken, BS; Storzbach, D. Effects of oxcarbazepine and phenytoin on the EEG and cognition in healthy volunteers. *Epilepsy and Behavior,* 2004, 5, 894-902.

[85] Aikia, M; Kalviainen R, Silvenius, J; Halonen, T; Riekkinen, PJ. Cognitive effects of oxcarbazepine and phenytoin monotherapy in newly diagnosed epilepsy: one year follow up. *Epilepsy Research,* 1992, 11(3), 199-203.

[86] Huang, C-W; Pai, M-C; Tsai, J-J. Comparative cognitive effects of levetiracetam and topiramate in intractable epilepsy. *Psychiatry and Clinical Neurosciences,* 2008, 548-553.

[87] Piazzini, A; Chifari, R; Canevini, MP; Turner, K; Fontana, SP; Canger, R. Levetiracetam: An improvement of attention and of oral fluency in patients with partial epilepsy. *Epilepsy Research,* 2006, 68, 181–188.

[88] Neyens, LGJ; Alpherts, WCJ; Aldenkamp, AP. Cognitive effects of a new pyrrolidine derivative (levetiracetam) in patients with epilepsy. *Progress in Neuropsychopharmacology and Biological Psychiatry*, 1995, 19, 411-419.

[89] Meador, KJ; Gevins, A; Loring, DW; McEvoy, LK; Ray, PG; Smith, ME; Motamedi, GK; Evans, BM; Baum, C. Neuropsychological and neurophysiologic effects of carbamazepine and levetiracetam. *Neurology,* 2007, 69, 2076-2084.

[90] Herranz, JL; Armijo, JA; Arteaga R. Clinical side effects of phenobarbital, primidone, phenytoin, carbamazepine, and valproate during monotherapy in children. *Epilepsia,* 1988, 29(6), 794-804.

[91] Stores, G. Behavioural effects of anti-epileptic drugs. *Developmental Medicine and Child Neurology*, 1975, 17(5), 647-58.

[92] Iivanianen, M; Savolainen, H. Side effects of Phenobarbital and phenytoin during long-term treatment of epilepsy. *Acta Neurologica Scandinavica,* 1983, 97, 49-67.

[93] Sher, A; Andersen, JM; Bhatia, SC. "Primidone-induced catatonic schizophrenia". *Drug Intelligence and Clinical Pharmacy* 1983, 17(7–8), 551–552.

[94] Mattson, RH; Cramer, JA; Collins, JF; Smith, DB; Delgado-Escueta, AV; Browne, TR; Williamson, PD; Treiman, DM; McNamara, JO; McCutchen, CB; et al. Comparison of carbamazepine, phenobarbital, phenytoin, and primidone in partial and secondarily generalized tonic-clonic seizures. *New England Journal of* Medicine 1985, 313(3), 145–151.

[95] Banu, SH; Jahan, M; Koli, UK; Ferdousi, S; Khan, NZ; Neville, B. Side effects of phenobarbital and carbamazepine in childhood epilepsy: randomized controlled trial. *British Medical Journal,* 2007, 334(7605), 1207.

[96] Pulliainen, V; Jokelainen, M. Effects of phenytoin and carbamazepine on cognitive functions in newly diagnosed epileptic patients. *Acta Neurologica Scandinavica,* 1994, 89(2), 81-86.

[97] Cramer, JA; Menachem, EB; French, J. Review of treatment options for refractory epilepsy: new medications and vagal nerve stimulation. *Epilepsy Research,* 2001, 47, 17-25.

[98] Perucca, E; Aldenkamp, A; Tallis, R; Kramer, G. Role of valproate across the ages. Treatment of epilepsy in the elderly. *Acta Neurologica Scandinavica,* 2006, 114(184), 28-37.

[99] Wilson, EA; Brodie, MJ. New anti-epileptic drugs. In: Brodie, MJ; Treiman, DM (Eds.). *Modern Management of Epilepsy.* London: Bailliere-Tindall, 1996.

[100] Camposano, SE; Major, P; Halpern, E; Thiele, EA. Vagabatrin in the treatment of childhood epilepsy: A retrospective chart review of efficacy and safety profile. *Epilepsia,* 2008, 49(7), 1186-1191.

[101] Sheth, RD; Buckley, D; Penney, S; Hobbs, GR. Vigabatrin in childhood epilepsy: Comparable efficacy for generalized and partial seizures. *Clinical Neuropharmacology,* 1996, 19(4), 297-304.

[102] Herranz, JL; Arteaga, R; Farr, IN; Valdizan, E; Beaumont, D; Armijo, JA. Dose-response study of vigabatrin in children with refractory epilepsy. *Journal of Child Neurology,* 1991, 6(S2), S45-S51.

[103] Turanli, G; Celebi, A; Yalnizoglu, D; Topcu, M; Anlar, B; Topaloglu, H; Aysun, S. Vigabatrin in pediatric patients with refractory epilepsy. *Turkish Journal of Pediatrics, 2006*, 48(1), 25-30.

[104] Guberman, A. Vigabatrin. *Canadian Journal of Neurological Sciences,* 1996, 23(4), S13-S17.

[105] Aldenkamp, AP; Vermeulen, J; Mulder, OG; Overweg, J; Vanparys, JAP; Beun, AM; Vantslot, B. Gamma-vinyl GABA (Vigabatrin) and mood disturbances. *Epilepsia,* 1994, 35(5), 999-1004.

[106] Morris, GL. Efficacy and tolerability of gabapentin in clinical practice. *Clinical Therapeutics,* 1995, 17(5), 891-900.

[107] Lee, DO; Steingard, RL; Cesena, M; Helmers, SL; Riviello, JJ; Mikati, MA. Behavioural side effects of gabapentin in children. *Epilepsia,* 1996, 37(1), 87-90.

[108] Harden, CL; Hosain, S; Nikolov, B; Labar, DR. Evaluation of Gabapentin in an Outpatient and Office-based Sample of Epilepsy Patients. *Journal of Epilepsy,* 1998, 11, 130-135.

[109] Rejis, R; Aldenkamp, AP; De Krom, M. Mood effects of anti-epileptic drugs. *Epilepsy and Behavior,* 2004, 5, S66-76.

[110] Jan, MMS; Zuberi, SA; Alsaihati, BA. Pregabalin: Preliminary Experience in Intractable Childhood Epilepsy. *Pediatric Neurology,* 2009, 40(5), 347-350.

[111] Lassen, LC; Sommerville, K; Mengel, HB; Edwards, D; Nielson, B; Shu, V. Summary of five controlled trials of tiagabine as adjunctive treatment of patients with partial seizures. *Epilepsia,* 1995, 36, S148.

[112] Sveinbjornsdottir, S; Sander, JW; Patsalos, PN; Upton, D; Thompson, PJ; Duncan, JS. Neuropsychological effects of tiagabine, a potential new antiepileptic drug. *Seizure,* 1994, 3, 29-35.

[113] Leppik, E. Tiagabine: the safety landscape. *Epilepsia,* 1995, 36, 10-13.

[114] Leppik, IE; Gram, L; Deaton, R; Sommerville, KW. Safety of tiagabine: summary of 53 trials. *Epilepsy Research,* 1999, 33, 235-246.

[115] Dichter, MA; Brodie, MJ. New anti-epileptic drugs. *New England Journal of Medicine*, 1996, 334, 1583-1590.

[116] Booth, F et al: Canadian Study Group for Chilhood Epilepsy. Clobazam Has Equivalent Efficacy to Carbamazepine and Phenytoin as Monotherapy for Childhood Epilepsy. *Epilepsia,* 1998, 39(9), 952-959.

[117] Mehndriatta, MM; Krishnamurthy, M; Rajesh, KN; Singh, G. Clobazam monotherapy in drug naive adult patients with epilepsy. *Seizure: European Journal of Epliepsy,* 2003, 12(4), 226-228.

[118] Jan, MM; Shaabat, AO. Clobazam for the treatment of intractable childhood epilepsy. *Saudi Medical Journal,* 2000, 21(7), 622-624.

[119] Mula, M; Trimble, MR. The importance of being seizure free: topiramate and psychopathology in epilepsy. *Epilepsy and Behavior,* 2003, 4, 430–434.

[120] Bootsma, HPR; Ricker, L; Diepman, L; Gehring, J; Hulsman, J; Lambrechts, D; Leenan, L; Majoie, M; Schellekens, A; de Krom, M; Aldenkamp, AP. Long-term effects of levetiracetam and topiramate in clinical practice. *Seizure,* 2008, 17, 19-26.

[121] Roberts, GMP; Majoie, HJM; Leenen, LAM; Bootsma, HP; Kessels, AGH; Aldenkamp, AP; Leonard, BE. Ketter's hypothesis of the mood effects of antiepileptic drugs coupled to the mechanism of action of topiramate and levetiracetam. *Epilepsy and Behavior*, 2005, 6(3), 366-372.

[122] Bootsma, HPR; Coolen, F; Aldenkamp, AP; Arends, J; Diepman, L; Hulsman, J; Lambrechts, D; Leenen, L; Majoie, M; Schellekens, A; de Krom, M. Topiramate in clinical practice: long-term experience in patients with refractory epilepsy referred to a tertiary epilepsy center. *Epilepsy and Behavior,* 2004, 5(3), 380-387.

[123] Stephens, LJ; Sills, GJ; Brodie, MJ. Topiramate in refractory epilepsy: A prospective observational study. *Epilepsia,* 2000, 41(8), 977-980.

[124] Mohamed, K; Appleton, R; Rosenbloom, L. Efficacy and tolerability of topiramate in childhood epilepsy: a clinical experience. *Seizure*, 2000, 9, 137-141.

[125] Al Ajlouni, S; Shorman, A; Daoud, AS. The efficacy and side effects of topiramate on refractory epilepsy in infants and young children: A multi-center clinical trial. *Seizure,* 2005, 14(7), 459-463.

[126] Kluger, G; Zsoter, A; Holyhausen, H. Long-term use of zonisamide in refractory childhood-onset epilepsy. *European Journal of Pediatric Neurology,* 2008, 12, 19-23.

[127] Seki, T; Kumagai, N; Maezawa, M. Effects of zonisamide monotherapy in children with epilepsy. *Seizure: European Journal of Epilepsy,* 2004, 13(S1), S26-S32.

[128] Hirari, K; Kimiya, S; Tabata, K; Seki, T; Jozaki, K; Kumagai, N. Selective mutism and obsessive compulsive disorders associated with zonisamide. *Seizure,* 2002, 11(7), 468-470.

[129] Mayahara, K; Kanemoto, K; Kawasaki, J; Nakagawa, Y; Nishikawa, S; Kawai, I. Zonisamide and episodic psychosis (in Japanese). *Journal of Japan Epilepsy Society,* 1995, 13, 177-183.

[130] Kimura, S. Zonisamide-induced behavior disorder in two children. *Epilepsia,* 1994, 35, 403-405.

[131] Miyamoto, T; Kohsaka, M; Koyama, T. Psychotic episodes during zonisamide treatment. *Seizure,* 2000, 9, 65-70.

[132] Aldenkamp, AP; Arends, J; Bootsma HP; Diepman, L; Hulsman, J; Lambrechts, D; Leenen, L; Majoie, M; Schellekens, A, de Vocht, J. Randomized, double-blind parallel-group study comparing cognitive effects of a low-dose lamotrigine with valproate and placebo in healthy volunteers. *Epilepsia,* 2002, 43, 19-26.

[133] Brodie, MJ; Richens, A; Yuen, AW. Double-blind comparison of lamotrigine and carbamazepine in newly diagnosed epilepsy: UK Lamotrigine/Carbamazepine Monotherapy and Trial Group. *Lancet,* 1995, 345, 476-479.

[134] Schapel, G; Chadwick, D. A survey comparing lamotrigine and vigabatrin in everyday clinical practice. *Seizure,* 1996, 5, 267-270.

[135] Calabrese, JR; Rapport, DJ; Shelton, MD; Kujawa, M; Kimmel, SE. Clinical studies on the use of lamotrigine in bipolar disorder. *Neuropsychobiology,* 1998, 38, 185-91.

[136] Green, B. Lamotrigine in mood disorders. *Current Medical Research Opinions,* 2003, 19, 272-277.

[137] Barron, TF; Hunt, SL; Hoban, TF; Price, ML. Lamotrigine monotherapy in children. *Pediatric Neurology,* 2000, 23(2), 160-163.

[138] Dogan, EA; Usta, BE; Bilgen, R; Senol, Y; Aktekin, B. Efficacy, tolerability, and side effects of oxcarbazepine monotherapy: A prospective study in adult and elderly patients with newly diagnosed partial epilepsy. *Epilepsy and Behavior,* 2008, 13, 156-161.

[139] Raju, GP; Sarco, DP; Poduri, A; Riviello, JJ; Bergin, AMR; Takeoka, M. Oxcarbazepine in children with nocturnal frontal-lobe epilepsy. *Pediatric Neurology,* 2007, 37, 345-349.

[140] Franzoni, E; Garone, C; Sarajlija, J; Gualandi, S; Malaspina, E; Cecconi, I; Moscano, FC; Marchiani, V. Open prospective study on oxcarbazepine in epilepsy in children: A preliminary report. *Seizure,* 2006, 15, 292-298.

[141] Besag, FM. Behavioural effect of the new anticonvulsants. *Drug Safety,* 2001, 24, 513-536.

[142] French, J; Edrich, P; Cramer, JA. A systematic review of the safety profile of levetiracetam: a new antiepileptic drug. *Epilepsy Research,* 2001, 47, 77-90.

[143] Schulze-Bonhage, A; Feil, B; Fauser, S; Homberg, V. Levetiracetam in combined therapy for focal epilepsy: experience with 80 patients. *Nervenartz,* 2004, 75(8), 749-754.

[144] Opp, J; Tuxhorn, I; May, T; Kluger, G; Wiemer-Kruel, A; Kurlemann, G; Gross-Selbeck, G; Rating, D; Brandl, U; Bettendorf, U; Hartel, C; Korn-Merker, E. Levetiracetam in children with refractory epilepsy: A multicenter open label study in Germany. *Seizure*, 2005, 14(7), 476-484.

[145] Cramer, JA; De Rue, K; Devinsky, O; Edrich, P; Trimble, MR. A systematic review of the behavioral effects of levetiracetam in adults with epilepsy, cognitive disorders, or an anxiety disorder during clinical trials. *Epilepsy and Behavior,* 2003, 4, 124-32.

[146] Bootsma, HPR; Ricker, L; Diepman, L; Gehring, J; Hulsman, J; Lambrechts, D; Leenen, L; Majoie, M; Schellekens, A; de Krom, M; Aldenkamp, AP. Levitiracetam in clinical practice: Long-term experience in patients with refractory epilepsy referred to a tertiary epilepsy center. *Epilepsy and Behavior,* 2007, 10, 296-303.

[147] Herranz, JL; Rufo-Campos, M; Arteaga, R. Effectiveness and tolerability of levetiracetam in 43 children and adolescents with epilepsy. *Revista de Neurologia,* 2003, 37(11), 1005-1008.

[148] Lagae, L; Buvse, G; Ceulemans, B. Clinical experience with levetiracetam in childhood epilepsy: an add-on and mono-therapy trial. *Seizure*, 2005, 14(1), 66-71.

[149] National Institute for Health and Clinical Excellence. *The epilepsies: the diagnosis and management of the epilepsies in adults and children in primary and secondary care.* London: NICE, 2004.

[150] Cavanna, AE; Monaco, F. Brain mechanisms of altered conscious states during epileptic seizures. *Nature Reviews Neurology,* 2009, 5, 267-276.

In: Seizures and Anti-Epileptic Drugs
Editors: Willard Hosten and Aleph Burtsev
ISBN: 978-1-62100-255-0

Chapter III

Epilepsy Related Injuries

Andrea N. Lees
Aged Care Department, Royal Hobart Hospital,
Tasmania, Australia

Abstract

Since 1960 there have been reports that those with epilepsy are more prone to injuries compared to those without epilepsy. The largest population-based study to date reported that persons with epilepsy were 1.4 times more likely to have sustained an injury for which medical attention was sought.

Risk factors for injuries have been reported to include seizure frequency, disease duration, treatment duration, cognitive handicap and seizure-type. Most of the seizure-types included in studies were tonic-clonic seizures and seizures causing falls. Seizures resulting in falls increase the risk of concussion and other injuries. Most recurrent seizure-related injuries involve head injury.

Most injuries are minor. However more serious injury rates are increased. The risk of fracture is elevated almost 2-fold, either resulting directly from seizure-induced injury or predisposed by drug-induced reduction in bone mineral density. Hip and femur fractures are the most common.

Submersion injury has a high mortality; the risk of submersion in people with epilepsy is 18.7 fold higher than in the general population.

Although population and prospective studies have reported no significant difference in burns between persons with epilepsy and those without, there are conflicting data.

The risk of motor vehicle accidents in drivers with epilepsy also appears increased, albeit marginally.

While it is appropriate to mandate appropriate restrictions to reduce injury, such as limitations on driving and certain sports or activities, excessive limitations may further limit achievement of independence. Appropriate vitamin D and calcium supplementation and periodic measurement of bone mineral density in those at risk for osteoporosis are recommended.

Introduction

People with epilepsy are considered to be at higher risk of incurring accidental injury than those without seizures. The World Health Organization (WHO) states that epilepsy accounts for 0.5% of the global burden of disease and 0.2% of total deaths [1]. Understanding injury types and frequency in persons with epilepsy is crucial, as injuries can affect quality of life, employability, and insurance eligibility, educational and recreational opportunities.

What Is the Evidence for Increased Injury?

Various studies have reported on accidental injury rates in cohorts with epilepsy (Table 1). These included studies from emergency room admissions [2], multicentre cohort studies [3], and population-based studies [2, 4-6]. One recent Canadian population-based study did not find an association between epilepsy and injury based on self-report [5]. Many of the studies, however, are not population-based, or are limited to certain age groups or to observing overall injuries, single injury type, or defining injury based on self-report. Many studies include no controls, and contextual comparisons are not possible.

The most robust data comes from the largest population-based study to date [6] which reported a 20.6% incidence of at least one injury among persons with epilepsy (N=8890) compared to 16.0% among those without epilepsy (N=26,670) ($p < 0.001$) over a 1-year period, in a large Canadian health region. The mean age was 37.4 years (range 0.01-96.4 years), and 51.3% of subjects were male. The study only captured those injuries where medical attention was sought, therefore presumably capturing more severe injuries. Those with epilepsy were 1.4 times more likely to have sustained an injury for which medical attention was sought after adjusting for age, sex, and co-morbidities. Persons with epilepsy were at a higher risk of fractures, crushing injuries, intracranial injuries, other types of head injury, and multiple injuries. Severity of epilepsy and injury were not considered in this study. Nor did this study determine if injuries were seizure-related.

The largest prospective investigation of this topic was done in a multicentre, European cohort of 951 children (aged more than 5 years) and adults with idiopathic, cryptogenic, remote symptomatic epilepsy followed prospectively for 17,484 person-months, and compared to a cohort of 909 matched controls [3, 7]. Cases were recruited from both general hospital and university settings and followed between 1 and 2 years. Children less than 5 years of age were excluded, as were those with acute or progressing epileptogenic conditions. Partial epilepsies accounted for 55% of the cohort and seizure frequency at study entry was less than monthly in 70%. Cases with epilepsy had a significantly higher cumulative probability of an accident than controls both at 12 (17% versus 12%, $p < 0.0001$) and 24 months (27% versus 17%, $p < 0.0001$). In the epilepsy group, 24% of accidents were seizure-related, but after exclusion of these there was no significant difference in the accident rate between cases with epilepsy and controls. However, further analysis did show that, even after controlling for seizure-related accidents, cases with epilepsy have a higher rate of domestic, street, and work accidents than controls. The overall injury rate was neither significantly correlated with seizure frequency nor aetiology. Most accidents were minor. However, cases with epilepsy reported higher rates of hospitalization (3% versus 1%) and medical action after an accident (16% versus 10%), compared to controls.

Although most studies have reported a higher rate of injuries in those with compared to those without epilepsy, there are conflicting data. For example, a Canadian population-based study [5] examined the 12-month frequency of injuries in those with epilepsy (n=835) compared to those without epilepsy (n=130047), using the door-to-door Canadian Community Health Survey (CCHS), a validated self-report questionnaire which targeted persons aged 12 years and older, living in private dwellings, and representing 98% of the Canadian population. A response rate of 85% was achieved. They found that the overall 12-month rate of injuries was not significantly different in those with epilepsy (14.9%) compared with the general population (13.3%). Several possible methodologic differences may explain this discrepancy. First, the CCHS relies on self-report and therefore can be associated with recall bias. Second, the CCHS excludes individuals in institutions, a population that may be at substantially higher risk of injuries and falls. The authors did not have exact estimates of the proportion of people with epilepsy who reside in institutions in Canada, but nevertheless surmised that the proportion would be small and therefore likely to have a small contribution to their estimates. Third, the CCHS asked specifically about injuries that were sufficiently severe to limit normal activities, and repetitive injuries were excluded.

However this study did show that among individuals reporting injuries, there was a significantly lower frequency of sports-related injuries in people with epilepsy (RR: 0.7, CI95:0.4-0.9). The large European study [3, 7] and other researchers have made similar observations [3, 8, 9]. A possible explanation includes lower levels of physical and certain sports activities among people with epilepsy because of concerns [10] of injuries during seizures [11].

The Canadian population-based study [5] also reported a three-times higher frequency of hospitalization following injuries in people with epilepsy (RR: 3.0, CI95:1.3-4.7) despite having no more severe injuries. This could reflect that hospitalization is related to seizures and to co-morbidities, and not injuries alone, or a more cautious attitude of clinicians towards injuries in people with epilepsy.

A population-based longitudinal retrospective non-controlled study in 247 Rochester residents diagnosed with epilepsy [12] similarly found that seizure-related injuries are infrequent and generally of minor severity. An inclusion criterion for that study was any injury resulting from a seizure, other than orolingual trauma, sufficient for the patient to seek medical attention. Sixteen percent of persons with epilepsy had seizure-related injuries (one injury in every 44 person-years), with most injuries (79%) being cranial soft-tissue contusions or lacerations (79%).

The literature concerning seizure-related injuries in childhood is limited. Childhood is an accident-prone age, and epilepsy might increase the likelihood of accidents during childhood.

Using a structured questionnaire, Appleton collected information on seizure-related injury in 198 children aged 1-16 years of age, presenting with two or more newly diagnosed, afebrile seizures at several centres in the United States and found seizure-induced injury to be uncommon [9]. Only 25 (12.6%) had experienced an injury prior to the diagnosis of epilepsy, with 4 of these requiring medical attention for this injury. Similar to previous studies, most injuries were seen in patients with tonic-clonic or myoclonic seizures.

Table 1. Key studies of injury rates in epilepsy

Author/year of publication	Type of design	Age of population	Key findings
Nakken and Lossius. (1993) [41]	Norwegian prospective, non-controlled.	21-82	32.3% of 62 multi handicapped adults sustained a seizure-related injury in a 13-month period
Kirby and Sadler (1995) [2]	Canadian prospective, non-controlled	>15	15% of seizures that presented to the emergency department resulted in injury or death
Buck et al (1997) [19]	UK retrospective non-controlled	>16	35% sustained a seizure-related injury over the prior 12 months
Neufeld et al. (1999) [8]	Retrospective survey of 298 adults in Israel with epilepsy regarding past injuries during seizures, epilepsy clinic	16-85	30% reported prior trauma with seizures
Kirsch and Wirrell (2001) [13]	Canadian retrospective controlled	5-16	No difference in prevalence of injuries between persons with or without epilepsy
Appleton (2002) [9]	UK prospective non-controlled	1-16	12.6% sustained an injury during a seizure before a diagnosis of epilepsy was established
Lawn et al. (2004) [12]	US retrospective, non-controlled	13-70	62 seizure-related injuries occurred in 39 persons (16% of the cohort, 1 in 44 person-years)
Van den Broek et al (2004) [3]	European prospective controlled	>/=5	At 2 years those with epilepsy were significantly more likely to have sustained an injury compared to those without epilepsy (21% vs 14%)
Souverein et al (2005) [4]	UK retrospective controlled	All ages	Incidence of fractures: persons with epilepsy 241.9/10,000 person years vs without epilepsy 123.5/10,000 person years.
Buffo et al (2008) [14]	Brazilian retrospective non-controlled	6 months-18yo	44% of the children with epilepsy had a seizure related accident; in 18% these caused injury severe enough to require a visit to the emergency room
Tellez-Zenteno et al (2008) [5]	Canadian retrospective controlled	>/=12	No difference in injury risk between persons with epilepsy (14.9%) and without epilepsy (13.3%)

Author/year of publication	Type of design	Age of population	Key findings
Kwon et al (2010) [6]	Canadian retrospective controlled	0.01-96.4	The 1 year incidence of overall injuries was 20.6% among persons with epilepsy and 16.1% among those without epilepsy (statistically significant)
Ting and Kwong (2010) [15]	Hong Kong retrospective non-controlled	<18	9% (11 of 122) children with newly diagnosed epilepsy had a seizure-related injury

Similarly, in a small case controlled study comparing cognitively normal children with epilepsy to age- and gender-matched controls, Kirsch found no increased rate of injury in those with epilepsy [13]. However, the small number of children with comorbid attention deficit disorder did have a higher rate of injury.

In contrast, a retrospective study by Buffo et al reported that 44% children with epilepsy at a Brazilian hospital paediatric clinic experienced seizure-related accidents [14]. One hundred consecutive children with epilepsy were evaluated using a structured questionnaire. Ages ranged from 6 months to 18 years old (mean =9years). Epilepsy was idiopathic in 14 patients, symptomatic in 51, and cryptogenic in 35. Developmental delay, however, was present in 51 patients. 18 patients needed medical assistance at an emergency room due to the injury from the seizure. This finding is alarming, especially because seizure related accidents happened at an age in which children often are supervised for most of the time. In 40 patients a seizure related accident was prevented by a bystander. Fourteen patients described situations where their seizures could have caused an accident, but where this was averted by good luck. Contusions and lacerations were the most common type of injury associated with seizures. Patients presenting with seizure related accidents were on a higher number of anti-epileptic drugs than those in which no accidents happened ($p<0.05$).

Ting et al [15] prospectively surveyed 122 children under the age of 18, with newly diagnosed epilepsy presenting to a Hong Kong hospital. Fifty-five (45.1%) patients were classified as manifesting idiopathic epilepsy, 25 (20.5%) as manifesting cryptogenic epilepsy, and 42 (34.4%) as manifesting symptomatic epilepsy. Patients with only febrile convulsions, acute symptomatic seizures, single seizures, and neonatal seizures were excluded. Children with seizure-related injuries were compared with those without injuries. The mean duration of follow-up was 26 months (range, 14-36 months). Most injuries occurred during the first seizure, before epilepsy was diagnosed, but most of the injuries were minor and occurred whilst asleep. After diagnosis, the number of injuries was remarkably small. Eleven (9%) children manifested 12 seizure-related injury episodes. Seventy-three percent of patients with injuries had normal neurodevelopmental status. Injury occurred at a mean age of 11.6 years, and epilepsy was diagnosed at a mean age of 13.8 years, in those with seizure-induced injuries. Injury occurred at first seizure presentation or upon diagnosis of epilepsy in 72.7% patients. Ten (90.9%) children were not receiving antiepileptic drugs at their time of injury. Children with generalized convulsions were at a significantly higher risk of seizure-related injuries: generalised tonic-clonic seizures accounted for 72.7% of seizure-related injuries and partial seizures accounted for 18.2% (odds ratio, 3.77; 95% CI 0.95-14.98; $p=0.045$).Soft-tissue and dental injuries comprised 91.7% and 75%, respectively, of injuries occurring at home. No seizure-related mortality occurred.

What Types of Injury Are most Concerning?

Submersion injuries, motor vehicle accidents, burns and head injuries are among the most feared epilepsy-related injuries [16]. However contusions and wounds are the most common injuries, followed by abrasions, fractures, brain concussions, sprains/strains and burns [17].

Submersion Injury

Submersion injury appears the most likely injury type that leads to death [18]. In a retrospective survey of adults in the United Kingdom, with at least one seizure in the previous 12 months, 44 of 313 (14%) reported sustaining a seizure while bathing or swimming in the preceding 12 months [19]. Patients having at least one seizure a month and those reporting at least 3 drug-related adverse effects were more likely than the rest to experience a seizure while bathing or swimming [19].

Five investigators in London, using meta-analytic methods, calculated standardized mortality ratios (SMRs) with 95% confidence intervals for 51 cohorts of people with epilepsy for whom the number of deaths by drowning could be estimated [20], and compared these with the total population by person-years at risk. Four point seven drowning deaths were expected for the general population in that time period, but 88 were observed in the epilepsy population, giving a huge SMR of 18.7. Further breakdown showed an SMR of 18 in prevalent epilepsy, 25.7 in epilepsy and learning disability, 41.1 in those who had been treated with temporal lobe excision, and 96.9 in those in institutional care.

The SMR for children, though both statistically and relevantly increased, was significantly smaller than adults (SMR 7.76 in children and 20.04 in adults, ratio 0.39 (CI95% 0.13-0.999)). This may be due to increased supervision of children with epilepsy in an age group in which the rate of drowning is generally the highest.

Similarly a retrospective survey from the United Kingdom found that children with epilepsy were 7.5 times more likely to experience submersion injury or death than those without seizures [21]. Of 306 children under the age of 15 who drowned or nearly drowned in the UK in 1988 and 1989, ten cases met the criteria of established epilepsy. All suffered tonic-clonic seizures and had been on anticonvulsant medication. Four of these children died. Five children had special needs. None of the children with primary epilepsy who were supervised at the time of the accident died, suggesting that if epileptic children are supervised they have no greater risk of a drowning death than the general population.

A retrospective, population-based cohort study of all submersion injuries in children and teens in a single county in Washington State, between 1974 and 1990, also noted a strikingly high risk of submersion injury in children with epilepsy. Of 336 submersions, 21 (6%) occurred among children with epilepsy. Relative risks were estimated using population-based estimates of epilepsy prevalence. Those with epilepsy had a relative risk of 13.9 for submersion, and 13.8 for fatal drowning compared to children without epilepsy, and were more likely to be 5 years of age or older at the time of injury (86% versus 47%). The most common sites for submersion were the bathtub or a swimming pool, with a relative risk of 96 for drowning in a bath, and of 23.4 for drowning in a pool [22].

Ryan also noted that most drownings in persons with epilepsy occurred in the bath, without direct supervision [23]. Of 482 deaths from drowning in Alberta from 1981 to 1990, 25 (5%) were directly related to seizures. Fifteen (60%) of the 25 deaths occurred while the person was taking a bath unsupervised. Only one person (4%) died whilst taking a shower. All the subjects were socially independent. The duration of the seizure disorder and the time since the last seizure were not helpful risk factors. Nineteen (83%) of 23 people who had been receiving anticonvulsant drug therapy had undetectable or subtherapeutic levels of one or more drugs at autopsy.

Burns

The occurrence of seizure-related burns as a source of admission to burns units has declined over the last three decades from 5-10 to 1.6% [24]. The burn size has also been found to decrease from 15 to 2% of the entire body surface [25]. In two large prospective studies and one large retrospective population-based study, patients with epilepsy were not at greater risk of burns than the general population [3, 6, 7]. As most burns occur during domestic activities, this decreasing trend has been interpreted as the consequence of a change from open flames to central heating. As traditionally women perform domestic activities, this could explain why women are twice as likely as men to be burnt [19]. Spitz et al. specifically investigated seizure-related burns [26] and reported that cooking on a stove was the most influential factor, followed by showering. Together with sex; severity and frequency of seizures [19], and total number of seizures during adult life [26] are key predictors of having a burn or scald.

Fractures

Epilepsy is associated with an increased risk of fractures, possibly due in part to seizure-related injuries and to antiepileptic drug-related bone loss [27, 28].

The largest study to date examined the risk of fractures in those with epilepsy (N=40,485) and without epilepsy (N=80,970) over an 8 year period [4]. They reported an increased fracture incidence in persons with compared to those without epilepsy (overall incidence rate of 241.9 per 10,000 person-years in persons with epilepsy compared to 123.5 per 10,000 person-years without). They found that the rate ratios were consistently elevated across subtypes, with the highest seen in hip and femur fractures (adjusted incidence density ratio = 2.8).

The 2-fold increase in fracture incidence is consistent with other retrospective studies. In the large population-based study reported by Kwon et al. [6], 326 (3.7%) of patients with epilepsy manifested a fracture compared with 564 (2.1%) of persons without epilepsy (OR adjusted for co-morbidities 1.8 (CI 95% 1.5-2.0)). Persson et al. [29] also looked at the risk of extremity fractures in 177 epilepsy outpatients and also reported a 2.4 times higher risk compared to regional rates (incidence rate of 23.8 per 1,000 person-years). Annegers et al.

[30] also observed a twofold increase in cadence of hip fractures in a cohort of 467 persons with epilepsy compared to the general population.

Table 2. Seizure related fractures in different epilepsy populations

Author/year of publication	Type of design	Key Findings
Annegers et al [30] (1989)	Retrospective, population-based review of fractures.	Hip fractures were 2.3-fold more common in patients with epilepsy.
Desai et al [35] (1996)	Retrospective review of fractures sustained in 185,066 seizures over 4,521 patient-years compared with 'normal' population.	4.3-fold increased risk for all fractures and 3.2 fold increased risk for fractures unrelated to seizures. Biggest risk for fractures of intertrochanteric region and ankle (9.9x for each).
Vestergaard et al [36] (1999)	Self-completed questionnaires on fractures completed by non institutionalised patients with epilepsy and randomly selected controls	Relative risk of fracture in those with epilepsy 2.0. Seizures accounted for 33.9% of all fractures in the epilepsy group
Persson et al [29] (2002)	Retrospective, neurology-clinic-based review of fractures in adults with epilepsy	Overall risk ratio of fracture in patients with epilepsy was 2.39. 43% of fractures were definitely or possibly seizure-related.
Van den Broek et al [3] (2004)	Prospective cohort of persons with epilepsy and non epileptic controls followed for 17,484 and 17,206 person-months, respectively	Relative risk of fracture in the epilepsy group:1.3 (95% CI 0.8-2.4)
Souverein et al [4] (2005)	Retrospective review of UK General Practice Research Database	Persons with epilepsy had an overall risk of fracture 1.89 times higher than controls, and risk of femur and hip fractures 2.79 times higher
Sheth et al [32] (2006)	Retrospective analysis of patients aged 10-90+, over a 7 year period at a single health centre in the USA. 750 people with epilepsy sustained fractures.	293 (39%) had pathological fractures and 457 (61%) had traumatic/seizure-related fractures. Fractures occurred in a bimodal age distribution, peaking in the fifth decade of life, followed by a smaller but important peak in the eighth decade.

Author/year of publication	Type of design	Key Findings
Gniatkowska-Nowakowska et al (2010) [34]	Polish controlled observational trial: 126 children with epilepsy aged 7-16 treated with antiepileptic drugs compared with 132 controls.	Frequency of fractures 2-3 times greater in children with epilepsy than in the control group.
Kwon et al [6] (2010)	1 year population-based Canadian study comparing the incidence and types of injuries in persons with and without epilepsy.	326 (3.7%) of patients with epilepsy manifested a fracture compared with 564 (2.1%) of persons without epilepsy (OR adjusted for co-morbidities 1.8 (CI 95% 1.5-2.0)).
Lees [31] (2010)	Retrospective review of seizure-related injuries in patients aged 65 years or older (N=19 seizure-related injuries) compared with 34 non-seizure–related injuries in the control group, in 1 Australian hospital	35% of seizure-related injuries were fractures. No significant difference with respect to fractures (P=0.06) between groups.

However in the only prospective study done to date, no increased risk of fractures was seen in persons with epilepsy (RR 1.3; CI 95% 0.8-2.4), although fractures did account for 11% of accidents in the epilepsy cohort [3].

Similarly, in the only study to evaluate injuries secondary to seizures in older people [31], there was no significant difference in the incidence of fractures compared to the control group. The author concluded that these findings suggest that falls rather than the seizures per se are the dominant influence in the pathogenesis of fractures in older persons with epilepsy.

Sheth et al [32] performed a retrospective analysis of 750 patients with epilepsy who sustained fractures over a seven year period. Among these patients, 293 (39%) had pathological fractures and 457 (61%) had traumatic/seizure-related fractures. Fractures occurred in a bimodal age distribution, peaking in the fifth decade of life, followed by a smaller but important peak in the eighth decade. The pathogenic mechanisms underlying fractures during these two peaks appear to be different. Traumatic/seizure-related mechanisms were the dominant influence in those <50 years old, whereas pathological fractures featured predominantly after this age. However 56% of all pathological fractures occurred in those <50 years of age. These findings appear to support the suggestion that epilepsy significantly shifts the expected age effect on fractures associated with osteopathies to younger than would be expected in the general population, where these fractures typically manifest in a more aged population [33]. Gender distribution in this cohort with fractures was significantly different. In those less than 50 years of age, males were much more likely to sustain a fracture compared with females. On the other hand, between the ages of 70 and 79, women were twice as likely as men to sustain fractures (11% versus 3.5%, P<0.02).

There are few studies in the literature regarding the characteristics of injuries sustained as a result of seizures in children. Gniatkowska-Nowakowska [34] observed 126 children with epilepsy aged 7-16 treated with antiepileptic drugs compared with 132 controls. The frequency of fractures was 2-3 times greater in the children with epilepsy than in the control group. Osteoporosis and osteopenia were also present in the children who had taken antiepileptic drugs. Differences in calcium and phosphate levels in blood and urine between study and control groups were also statistically significant ($P<0.001$).

Head Injuries

Most head traumas in patients with epilepsy are minor and are a frequent complication of seizures [8, 12]. In a prospective study of 298 adults with chronic, long-term epilepsy, 27,934 seizures were recorded, 45.2% of which were associated with falls [37]. A total of 766 head injuries resulted, 45% of which required suturing. Only three more serious head injuries occurred, one with skull fracture and one each with extradural and subdural haemorrhage.

In the large population-based study reported by Kwon et al. [6] head injuries were the most common type of injuries, including head (skull and facial) fractures (OR 2.6, 95% CI 1.6-4.2), head injury (others-including crushing injury, wound, superficial injury, injury to blood vessels and nerves) (OR 2.2, 95% CI 1.9-2.5) and intracranial injuries (OR 1.7, 95% CI 1.3-2.3). Other studies have also confirmed head injuries to be the most common site of injury [2, 8, 19]. The European prospective cohort study found that concussion was significantly more common than in controls (RR 2.6, 95% CI 1.2-5.8) [3]. Hauser et al [38] found that the number of head injuries observed in those with epilepsy in an urban community was increased threefold over that expected in those without epilepsy, although the prevalence of epilepsy was found to be higher than what was expected from prior studies.

Other studies have reported higher rates of serious injury, but are derived from highly selected populations. In a prospective cohort of 22 adults with head injuries resulting from falls due to seizures admitted to a neurosurgical service over an 8-year period, intracranial hematomas were present in 20 (91%), 18 of whom required neurosurgical evacuation [39]. Most recurrent seizure-related injuries (72%) involve head injury [40].

Soft Tissue Injuries

In the prospective European cohort study, contusions, wounds and abrasions accounted for 26%, 23%, and 11% of accidents in persons with epilepsy [3] and all of these injury types were more prevalent in the cohort with epilepsy than controls. In all cases, once seizure-related events were excluded, there were no significant differences between cases and controls. Five percent of cases required medical attention following a contusion and 4% following a wound. In a prospective study of multi-handicapped patients with seizures, soft-tissue injuries accounted for 59 out of 80 (74%) seizure-related injuries [41].

In the only study to evaluate injuries secondary to seizures in older people [31], the most common injuries were soft tissue injuries (55%) and fractures (35%). The study group had significantly more soft tissue injuries without lacerations than the control group ($P=0.002$) but for soft tissue injuries with lacerations there was no significant difference ($P=0.41$) between cases and controls. Similarly, in children, soft tissue injuries appear to be the most common seizure-related injury [14, 15].

In a retrospective study of 33 children who had been prescribed helmets for intractable seizures resulting in falls, Deekollu et al. documented a seizure-related injury risk of 0.4%; scalp and facial bruises and lacerations were the most commonly seen injury type [42]. Interestingly, in this study, helmets did not appear to reduce the risk of facial or scalp injury – 21 of 31 (68%) of accidents occurring when a helmet was worn versus 16 of 28 (57%) of those seen when a helmet was not worn resulted in injuries to the face and scalp.

Dental Injuries

Not all studies have looked specifically at dental injury. In one retrospective survey of 975 adults with seizures, 9.7% of patients reported sustaining a dental injury as the result of a seizure, and in 86% of these cases, the injury resulted in either loss of teeth or fracture of the jaw [19]. Using questions similar to those utilised in a prior study [19], 52 consecutive adults treated with treatment-resistant epilepsy in New York, reported a total of 42 injuries [43]. Of these, 3 (7%) were dental injuries, all seizure-related, and of mild-moderate severity, as per Annegers et al classification scale [44].

In a prospective study of multi-handicapped adults with epilepsy, dental injuries accounted for only 4 of 80 (5%) seizure-related accidents [41].

One of the studies to specifically investigate dental injury [45] found that dental injury occurred in only 14 of the 1673 (1%) patients entered onto the Gloucestershire Epilepsy Database. However dental injury occurs significantly more often in patients with juvenile myoclonic epilepsy (JME), where it occurs in about 10%, most frequently involving injury to the front teeth.

In comparison, a Brazilian study of 109 consecutive patients with refractory epilepsy (mean age 38.81 +/- 14 years) reported 89 dental and oral injuries affecting 40.74% of patients. The subjects were interviewed using a dental questionnaire about frequency and type of orofacial injury during their lifetime. Subsequent to the interview, the patients were clinically examined.

The majority of injuries were crown fractures (42 subjects), followed by mandibular fractures (8 subjects) and tooth avulsion (eight subjects). Sixteen patients had more than 2 fractured teeth. The number of fractured teeth was associated with seizure frequency ($r2=0.59$, $P<0.001$), but was similar in patients with either temporal or extra-temporal epilepsy (0.53+/- 0.7 vs 0.73+/- 1.5, $P=0.43$) [46].

Dental injury has been reported in a series from Nigeria where 56 consecutive patients with epilepsy were reviewed by a dentist [47]. They found that 26 patients (46%) had traumatic anterior dental injury which they attributed to the traditional practice of forcing spoons and other hard objects between the teeth of patients during seizures [47].

Children with epilepsy are also at an increased risk of anterior tooth trauma [48, 49]. A study of 39 children with intractable epilepsy attending the UK National Centre for Young People with Epilepsy reported that 54% in all had experienced anterior tooth trauma, compared with the controls, 12.5% ($P<0.0001$) [48].

In a Turkish study, of 211 children with epilepsy, 58 (27.5%) had traumatised anterior teeth, which was reported as being higher than the control group, although exact figures were not reported [49].

Motor Vehicle Accidents

Many studies confirm that epilepsy poses some driving risk [50-54], but that risk seems limited and relatively small, particularly compared with alcohol [54-6]. For instance, one study estimated that the percentage of fatal driver crashes caused by a seizure is only 0.2% (86 of the total 44,027 annual driving fatalities in the US for the years 1995-1997) as compared with 30% caused by alcohol [54]; other studies concur that seizures pose a relatively low risk for fatal crashes [55-6]. Most investigations have demonstrated that the risk for any type of crash is estimated to be two-fold higher for people with epilepsy than for the general population [57-9]. However the risk level was determined based on crashes for all causes rather than just seizure-related crashes, which ought to be the most relevant concern in licensing drivers with epilepsy. In fact, in a population-based, retrospective cohort study of 30,420 licensed drivers, both with and without epilepsy in a regional area, it was reported that only 11% of all car crashes involving individuals with epilepsy are due to seizures [59]. Indeed, most car accidents involving people with epilepsy are not caused by a seizure but are due to driver error, just as occurs in the majority of crashes in the general population [57-9].

Although it is generally accepted that the seizure-free interval is a key determinant for licensing drivers [52], the exact duration of the legally required seizure-free interval is the subject of considerable debate [55-6, 60-2]. Krauss et al performed a retrospective case-control study comparing 50 patients with epilepsy who were involved in motor vehicle accidents during a seizure and 50 age- and gender-matched controls with epilepsy who had not crashed [52]. Groups were comparable for hours of driving per month and total years of driving. Adherence to a 12 month seizure-free interval was estimated to prevent about 80% of all crashes associated with seizures, but it would also prohibit driving for about 50% of all those with epilepsy who would not crash. In contrast, a 3 month seizure-free requirement prevents 50% of crashes but prohibits driving for only 25% of individuals who would not crash. However one study found that a 3 month seizure-free interval did not significantly increase the incidence of car crashes and deaths from seizures in the 3 years following implementation, as compared with a 1-year seizure-free requirement [63]. Another report found no difference in driver fatalities in states with short (ie 3 months) as compared with longer (ie 6- or 12-months) seizure-free requirements [54]. Although the key measure in determining licensure, the seizure-free interval is only one factor to be considered in setting standards. Factors significantly correlated with a lower rate of crashes include reliable auras with every seizure (OR 0.077), recent reduction or change in antiepileptic drugs (OR 0.111), and a previous history of fewer non-seizure-related accidents (OR 0.465) [52]. Another study reported that the risks are highest with a history of multiple seizures and in those not treated with antiepileptic drugs [64].

People who have had a single unprovoked seizure (which by definition does not constitute epilepsy) in the UK are allowed to regain their ordinary (group 1) driving licence 6 months after the event provided their risk of a seizure recurrence in the next year is below 20%. In a UK study 317 patients were randomised to immediate antiepileptic drug treatment, and 320 were deferred antiepileptic treatment [65]. In the immediate treatment group the unadjusted risk of recurrence in the next 12 months at 6 months after the index seizure was 14% (95%CI 10% to 18%), significantly below 20%. For the delayed treatment group the estimate was 18% (95%CI 13% to 23%) did not exclude a 20% risk of recurrence. At 12 months, however, the risk was reduced to 10% (95%CI 6% to 15%). Multivariate analyses identified subgroups with significantly greater than 20% risk of seizure recurrence in the 12 months after a six month seizure-free period, such as those with an abnormal electroencephalogram result and brain imaging; and, surprisingly, seizures whilst asleep.

In a study of risk factors for traffic accidents, Krauss et al noted that only 36% of patients with epilepsy had reported their seizures to the motor vehicle registry [52]. In addition, 54% of people involved in traffic accidents were found to be driving illegally. Likewise, nearly one third of patients with refractory partial epilepsy presenting for surgical evaluation were found to drive, with 26% reporting at least one accident owing to a seizure [66]. Of 245 adult persons with epilepsy in Thailand, 69 cases (28%) had a seizure whilst driving. Over half (36/69; 57%) had a seizure-related accident, most of which were mild but about 20% required hospitalization. Persons with epilepsy who had a seizure attack whilst driving had a significantly lower QOL in four of the eight categories of the SF-36 questionnaire [67].

Where do Injuries Occur?

Domestic, street and work accidents are, in decreasing order, the most common places for such injuries to occur [3,8-9], likely at least in part, due to time spent at home versus at other locations. This is not significantly different to the general population [5]. Studies on accidents at work in patients with epilepsy are scarce, and the evidence that epilepsy carries an increased risk of accidents at work is mostly anecdotal. In the European cohort study, the risk of accidents was approximately two-times higher in patients with idiopathic or remote symptomatic epilepsy than in the general population [3]. However, injuries were mostly mild and, with few exceptions, unrelated to seizures.

What Risk Factors Predispose to Injury?

Several factors predispose to a higher risk of injury among those with epilepsy. Seizure type has been a factor in most studies. Patients with generalised onset seizures, particularly tonic-clonic, atonic, or myoclonic seizures leading to falls, are at higher risk of concussion [3] as well as other injuries [8-9, 19]. Higher seizure frequency [3, 12, 19, 41], lack of a prolonged seizure-free interval [52], co-morbid attention deficit disorder, or cognitive handicap [22] may also increase the risk of injury. Therefore injury risk is not the same in all patients.

What Are Reasonable Recommendations to Minimize Injury Risk and Maximize Independence and Social Development?

While some restrictions are necessary to protect both the patient's and public's safety, restrictions themselves further limit independence and social development. Carpey et al. found that parents reported disability due to restrictions in 83% of children with active epilepsy [68]. Higher disability was seen in children whose neurologist had recommended at least some restrictions, emphasizing that physicians need to be aware of the impact of their recommendations when they counsel patients.

Seizure-related drownings represent a small but potentially preventable proportion of all drownings. Enhanced seizure control and compliance with anticonvulsant drug therapy may prevent some of these deaths. It is imperative that people with epilepsy and their families are appropriately counselled and the risk associated with activities explained to them. All people with epilepsy should be encouraged to shower in a non-glass cubicle, whilst sitting, rather than have a bath when possible. If bathing, the person with epilepsy should be seated in the bath, with the plug out. A hand-held shower head is recommended, whereby the flow of water can be cut off upon release of the instrument to prevent the tub from filling if the person blocks the drain during a seizure. The bathroom should remain unlocked. Bath time supervision of a young child with epilepsy is essential. A parent with epilepsy should be accompanied while bathing her/his baby or toddler [22, 23].

Swimming should only be permitted in restricted areas under the close supervision of a lifeguard who is well trained in cardiopulmonary resuscitation. In addition the lifeguard should be made aware of a person's epileptic condition. Children who have a fit in water disappear below the surface quickly and silently during the tonic phase of a fit [69]. Personal flotation devices should be worn at all times during boating activities. Risk-taking behaviour, for example alcohol, should be avoided [23].

Most burns/scalds occur with activities of daily living, and most of these can be avoided with improved safety measures that aid in preventing injury such as fire-resistant fabrics and furniture, radiator, fire and cooker guards, use of microwave ovens rather than stovetop cookers, installing thermostats to control water temperature, and keeping to a minimum the use of electric irons and hand-held hair dryers [26, 70].

Currently no consensus exists for screening, let alone the prevention and/or treatment of antiepileptic drug (AED)-induced bone loss [71-3]. Until such guidelines are developed, clinicians should follow recommendations put forth by the National Osteoporosis Foundation [74]. Lifestyle factors should be optimized, that is sunlight exposure and weight-bearing exercise as well as avoidance of risk factors such as bone-depleting drugs other than AEDs, smoking and heavy alcohol consumption [75]. Fall prevention strategies should be introduced as appropriate and good seizure control is important [76]. Enzyme inducing drugs and valproate should be avoided, if possible [71]. Appropriate vitamin D and calcium supplementation and periodic measurement of bone mineral density in those at risk for osteoporosis are recommended. It is not clear if bisphosphonates are effective in treating bone disorders in epilepsy [71].

While protective helmets are often recommended for this population, there have been few studies on the subject. Deekollu et al noted a high proportion of injuries even when helmets were worn [77]. Further work is needed to find a helmet design that is well tolerated and is effective at prevention of injury.

There is a need to create dental awareness in patients with epilepsy in order to improve their quality of life regarding aesthetics and orofacial function [46].

Driving as a quality of life issue should be discussed with patients. In determining appropriate driving restrictions for national guidelines, public safety must be balanced with the employment, social, and psychological impact to the individual with seizures. A good public transportation system would ease the need to drive.

Conclusion

Although people with epilepsy are at an increased risk of accidents and injuries, the majority of injuries are minor, and are mostly caused by an epileptogenic condition, an associated handicap or the recurrence of seizures. Associated handicaps and co-morbidity, where present, as well as antiepileptic drugs, may cause accidents and injuries by impairing cognitive functions and increasing the patient's susceptibility to suffer from the complications of injuries.

Contusions and sprains are the most common injuries, followed by abrasions, fractures, brain concussions, sprains/strains and burns. Patients with epilepsy are also at a higher risk of accidental death than the general population: submersion injury has a high mortality, whilst the risk of motor vehicle accidents is only marginally increased.

Accurate information, derived from studies, can assist in developing counselling strategies for patient safety and injury prevention strategies.

References

[1] Mathers C, Boerma T, Ma Fat D. (2008) *The global burden of disease in 2004.* Switzerland: WHO Press; 2008; 56, 62.

[2] Kirby S, Sadler RM. (1995) Injury and death as a result of seizures. *Epilepsia* 36:25-8.

[3] Van den Broek M, Beghi E; REST-1 Group. (2004) Accidents in patients with epilepsy: types, circumstances, and complications: a European cohort study. *Epilepsia* 45:667-72.

[4] Souverein PC, Webb DJ, Petri H, Weil J, Van Staa TP, Egberts T. (2005) Incidence of fractures among epilepsy patients: a population-based retrospective cohort study in the General Practice Research Database. *Epilepsia* 46:304-10.

[5] Tellez-Zenteno JF, Hunter G, Wiebe S. (2008) Injuries in people with self-reported epilepsy: a population-based study. *Epilepsia* 49:954-61.

[6] Kwon CS, Liu M, Quan H, Wiebe S, McChesney J, Wirrell E, Hamiwka L, Jette N. (2010) The incidence of injuries in persons with and without epilepsy – A population-based study. *Epilepsia* 51 (11):2247-53.

[7] Beghi E, Cornaggia C. (2004) Morbidity and accidents in patients with epilepsy: results of a European cohort study. *Epilepsia* 45:71-6.

[8] Neufeld MY, Vishne T, Chistik V, Korczyn AD. (1999) Life-long history of injuries related to seizures. *Epilepsy Res* 34:123-7.

[9] Appleton RE. (2002) Seizure-related injuries in children with newly diagnosed and untreated epilepsy. *Epilepsia* 43:764-7.

[10] Wolf P, Trimble MR. (1985) Biological antagonism and epileptic psychosis. *Br J Psychiatry* 146:272-6.

[11] Steinhoff BJ, Neususs K, Thegeder H, Reimers CD. (1996) Leisure time activity and physical fitness in patients with epilepsy. *Epilepsia* 37:1221-7.

[12] Lawn ND, Bamlet WR, Radhakrishnan K, O'Brien PC, So EL. (2004) Injuries due to seizures in persons with epilepsy: a population-based study. *Neurology* 63:156-70.

[13] Kirsch R, Wirrell E. Do cognitively normal children with epilepsy have a higher rate of injury than their nonepileptic peers? (2001) *J Child Neurol* 16:100-4.

[14] Buffo TH, Guerreiro MM, Tai P, Montenegro MA. (2008) Seizure-related accidents and injuries in childhood. *Arq Neuropsiquiatr* 66:458-61.
[15] Ting YW, Kwong KL. (2010) Seizure-related injuries in newly diagnosed childhood epilepsy. *Pediatr Neurol* 42:417-21.
[16] Tomson T, Beghi E, Sundqvist A, Johannessen SI. (2004) Medical risks in epilepsy: a review with focus on physical injuries, mortality, traffic accidents and their prevention. *Epilepsy Res* 60:1-16.
[17] Beghi E. (2009) Accidents and injuries in patients with epilepsy. *Expert Rev Neurother* 9(2):291-8.
[18] Wirrell EC. (2006) Epilepsy-related injuries. *Epilepsia* 47 (Suppl. 1):79-86.
[19] Buck D, Baker GA, Jacoby A, Smith DF, Chadwick DW. (1997) Patients' experiences of injury as a result of epilepsy. *Epilepsia* 38:439-44.
[20] Bell GS, Gaitatzis A, Bell CL, Johnson AL, Sander JW. (2008) Drowning in people with epilepsy: how great is the risk. *Neurology* 71:578-82.
[21] Kemp AM, Silbert JR. (1993) Epilepsy in children and the risk of drowning. *Arch Dis Child* 68:684-5.
[22] Diekema DS, Quan L, Holt VL. (1993) Epilepsy as a risk factor for submersion injury in children. *Pediatrics* 91:612-6.
[23] Ryan CA, Dowling G. (1993) Drowning deaths in people with epilepsy. *CMJA* 148:781-4.
[24] Josty IC, Narayanan V, Dickson WA. (2000) Burns in patients with epilepsy. Changes in epidemiology and implications for burn treatment and prevention. *Epilepsia* 41: 453-6.
[25] Richards EH. (1968) Aspects of epilepsy and burns. *Epilepsia* 9:127-35.
[26] Spitz MC, Towbin JA, Shantz D, Adler LE. (1994) Risk factors for burns as a consequence of seizures in persons with epilepsy. *Epilepsia* 35:764-7.
[27] Ensrud KE, Walczak TS, Blackwell TL, Ensrud ER, Bowman PJ, Stone KL. (2004) Antiepileptic drug use increase rate of bone loss in older women: a prospective study. *Neurology* 62:2051-7.
[28] Ensrud KE, Walczak TS, Blackwell TL, Ensrud ER, Barrett-Connor E, Orwoll ES. (2008) Antiepileptic drug use and rates of hip bone loss in older men: a prospective study. *Neurology* 71:723-30.
[29] Persson HB, Alberts KA, Farahmand BY, Tomson T. (2002) Risk of extremity fractures in adult outpatients with epilepsy. *Epilepsia* 43:768-72.
[30] Annegers JF, Melton LJ III, Sun CA, Hauser WA. (1989) Risk of age-related fractures in patients with unprovoked seizures. *Epilepsia* 30:348-55.
[31] Lees A. (2010) Retrospective study of seizure-related injuries in older people: A 10-year observation. *Epilepsy Behav* 19:441-4.
[32] Sheth RD, Gidal BE, Hermann BP. (2006) Pathological fractures in epilepsy. *Epilepsy Behav* 9:601-5.
[33] Ramsay RE, Rowan AJ, Pryor FM. (2004) Special considerations in treating the elderly patient with epilepsy. *Neurology* 62:S24-9.
[34] Gniatkowska-Nowakowska A. (2010) Fractures in epilepsy children. *Seizure* 19(6): 324-5.
[35] Desai KB, Ribbans WJ, Taylor GJ. (1996) Incidence of five common fracture types in an institutional epileptic population. *Injury* 27:97-100.

[36] Vestergaard P, Tigaran S, Rejnmark L, Tigaran C, Dam M, Mosekilde L. (1999) Fracture risk is increased in epilepsy. *Acta Neurol Scand* 99:269-75.

[37] Russell-Jones DL, Shorvon SD. (1989) The frequency and consequences of head injury in epileptic seizures. *J Neurol Neurosurg* Psychiatry 52:659-62.

[38] Hauser WA, Tabaddor K, Factor P, Finer C. (1984) Seizures and head injury in a urban community. *Neurology* 34:746-51.

[39] Zwimpfer TJ, Brown J, Sullivan I, Moulton RJ. (1997) Head injuries due to falls caused by seizures: a group at high risk for traumatic intracranial hematomas. *J Neurosurg* 86:433-7.

[40] Friedman DE, Tobias RS, Akman CI, O'Brian Smith E, Levin HS. (2010) Recurrent seizure-related injuries in people with epilepsy at a tertiary epilepsy center: A 2-year longitudinal study.

[41] Nakken KO, Lossius R. (1993) Seizure-related injuries in multi-handicapped patients with therapy-resistant epilepsy. *Epilepsia* 34:836-40.

[42] Deekollu D, Besag FM, Aylett SE. (2005) Seizure-related injuries in a group of young people with epilepsy wearing protective helmets: incidence, types and circumstances. *Seizure* 14:347-53.

[43] Friedman DE, Gilliam FG. (2010) Seizure-related injuries are underreported in pharmacoresistant localization-related epilepsy. *Epilepsia* 51(1):43-7.

[44] Annegers JF, Grabow JD, Groover RV, Laws ER Jr, Elveback LR, Kurland LT. (1980) Seizures after head trauma: a population study. *Neurology* 30:683-9.

[45] Thomas RH, Higgins S, Fuller GN. (2009) Dental injury during seizures associated with juvenile myoclonic epilepsy. *J Neurol Neurosurg* Psychiatry 80:91-3.

[46] Costa AL, Yasuda CL, Franca Jr MC, Morita ME, Cendes F. (2011) Refractory epilepsy is highly associated with severe dentoalveolar and maxillofacial injuries. *Epileptic Disord* Mar10 [Epub ahead of print].

[47] Ogunbodede EO, Adamolekun B, Akintomide AO. (1998) Oral health and dental treatment needs in Nigerian patients with epilepsy. *Epilepsia* 39:590-4.

[48] Percival T, Aylett SE, Pool F, Bloch-Zupan A, Roberts GJ, Lucas VS. (2009) *Eur Arch Paediatr Dent* Jan;10(1):19-24.

[49] Gurbuz T, Tan H. (2010) Oral health status in epileptic children. *Pediatr Int.* 52(2): 279-83.

[50] Gastaut H, Zifkin BG. (1987) The risk of automobile accidents with seizures occurring while driving: Relation to seizure type. *Neurology* 37:1613-6.

[51] Taylor J, Chadwick D, Johnson T. (1996) Risks of accidents in drivers with epilepsy. *J Neurol Neurosurg Psychiatry* 60:621-7.

[52] Krauss GK, Krumholz A, Carter RC, Kaplan P. (1999) Risk factors for seizure-related motor vehicle crashes in patients with epilepsy. *Neurology* 52:1324-9.

[53] Berg AT, Vickrey BG, Sperling MR, Langfitt JT, Bazil CW, Shinnar S, Parcia S, Spencer SS. (2000) Driving in adults with refractory localization-related epilepsy. Multi-center study of epilepsy surgery. *Neurology* 54:625-30.

[54] Sheth SG, Krauss G, Krumholz A, Li G. (2004) Mortality in epilepsy: Driving fatalities vs. other causes of death in patients with epilepsy. *Neurology* 63:1002-7.

[55] Krumholz A, Fisher RS, Lesser RP, Hauser WA. (1991) Driving and epilepsy: A review and reappraisal. *JAMA* 265:622-6.

[56] American Academy of Neurology, American Epilepsy Society, Epilepsy Foundation of America. Consensus statements, sample statutory provisions, and model regulations regarding driver licensing and epilepsy. (1994) *Epilepsia* 35:696-705.
[57] Waller JA. (1965) Chronic medical conditions and traffic safety. *N Eng J Med* 273:1413-20.
[58] Crancer A Jr, McMurray L. (1968) Accident and violation rates in Washington's medically restricted drivers. *JAMA* 205:74-9.
[59] Hansotia P, Broste SK. (1991) The effect of epilepsy or diabetes on the risk of automobile accidents. *N Eng J Med* 324:22-6.
[60] Krumholz A. (1994) Driving and epilepsy: a historical perspective and review of current regulations. *Epilepsia* 35:668-74.
[61] Krauss GK, Ampaw L, Krumholz A. (2001) Individual state driving restrictions for people with epilepsy in the US. *Neurology* 57:1780-5.
[62] Krumholz A. (2009) Driving issues in epilepsy: Past, present and future. *Epilepsy Curr* 9(2):31-5.
[63] Drazkowski JF, Fisher RS, Sirven JI, Demaerschalk BM, Uber-Zak L, Hentz JG, Labine D. (2003) Seizure-related motor vehicle crashes in Arizona before and after reducing the driving restriction from 12 to 3 months. *Mayo Clin Proc* 78:819.
[64] Hansotia P, Broste SK. (1993) Epilepsy and traffic safety. *Epilepsia* 34: 852-8.
[65] Bonnett LJ, Tudur-Smith C, Williamson PR, Marson AG. (2010) Risk of recurrence after a first seizure and implications for driving: further analysis of the Multicentre study of early Epilepsy and Single Seizures. *BMJ* 341:c6477.
[66] Berg AT, Vickrey BG, Sperling MR, Langfitt JT, Bazil CW, Shinnar S, Walczak TS, Pacia S, Spencer SS. (2000) Driving in adults with refractory localization-related epilepsy. *Neurology* 54:625-30.
[67] Tiamkao S, Sawanyawisuth K, Towanabut S, Visudhipun P, Thai QOL Epilepsy Investigators. (2009) *Can J Neurol Sci* 36(4):475-9.
[68] Carpey HA, Vermeulen J, Stroink H, Brouwer OF, Peters AC, van Donselaar CA, Aldenkamp AP, Arts WF. (1997) Disability due to restrictions in childhood epilepsy. *Dev Med Child Neurol* 39:521-6.
[69] Orlowski JP, Rothner AD, Leuders H. (1982) Submersion accidents in children with epilepsy. *Am J Dis Child* 136:777-80.
[70] Turner C, Spinks A, McClure R, Nixon J. (2004) Community-based interventions for the prevention of burns and scalds in children. *Cochrane Database Syst Rev* 3:CD004335.
[71] Sheth RD, Harden CL. (2007) Screening for bone health in epilepsy. *Epilepsia* 48(Suppl. 9):39-41.
[72] Trevathan E. (2008) Epilepsy-associated bone mineral density loss should be prevented. *Neurology* 70(3):166-7.
[73] Elliott J. (2009) Possible methods for the prevention of bone loss in persons with epilepsy. *Expert Rev Neurother* 9(6):797-812.
[74] Dawson-Hughes B; national Osteoporosis Foundation Guide Committee. (2008) A revised clinician's guide to the prevention and treatment of osteoporosis. *J Clin Endocrinol Metab* 93(7):2463-5.
[75] Nakken KO, Tauboll E. (2010) Bone loss associated with use of antiepileptic drugs. *Expert Opin Drug Saf* 9(4):561-71.

[76] Petty SJ, O'Brien TJ, Wark JD. (2007) Anti-epileptic medication and bone health. *Osteoporosis Int* 18:129-42.

[77] Deekollu D, Besag FM, Aylett SE. (2005) Seizure-related injuries in a group of young people with epilepsy wearing protective helmets: incidence, types and circumstances. *Seizure*. 14(5):347-53.

In: Seizures and Anti-Epileptic Drugs
Editors: Willard Hosten and Aleph Burtsev
ISBN: 978-1-62100-255-0

Chapter IV

Clinical Pharmacokinetic Characteristics of Novel Antiepileptic Drugs

Katarina Vučićević*[1]*, Branislava Miljković*[1]*,
***Sandra Vezmar Kovačević*[1]*, Zoran Todorović*[2] *and Milica Prostran*[2]**
[1]Department of Pharmacokinetics and Clinical Pharmacy,
Faculty of Pharmacy, University of Belgrade, Belgrade, Serbia
[2]Department of Pharmacology, Clinical Pharmacology and Toxicology,
School of Medicine, University of Belgrade, Belgrade, Serbia

Abstract

The choice of an antiepileptic drug (AED) is usually based upon the epileptic seizure type. However, pharmacokinetic (PK) characteristics of AEDs may be valuable support in choosing the optimal therapeutic option for the individual patient. The novel (second and third generation) AEDs include: eslicarbazepine acetate, felbamate, gabapentin, lacosamide, lamotrigine, levetiracetam, oxcarbazepine, pregabalin, rufinamide, stiripentol, tiagabine, topiramate, vigabatrin, and zonisamide. Although, these drugs belong to the same group, their individual PK characteristics differ. Gabapentin, unlike other new AEDs, is characterised by dose-dependent absorption, which is presumably caused by saturable L-amino acid transport system, and therefore its bioavailability ranges from 35-60%. Furthermore, gabapentin, pregabalin and vigabatrin are eliminated completely, while levetiracetam and topiramate are eliminated predominantly through the renal system. Therefore, PK variability of these individual drugs is less pronounced and more predictable in comparison to older AEDs. Their potential for drug interactions is minor, and consequently they have major clinical importance for patients with impaired hepatic function. On the other hand, felbamate, lamotrigine, oxcarbazepine, tiagabine and zonisamide are eliminated via metabolic pathways, either cytochrome P (CYP) 450, or conjugation dependent transformation. Oxcarbazepine is a prodrug, and its active metabolite is licarbazepine. These drugs interact with other drugs, and disease conditions, which alter the activity of metabolic enzymes; thus these changes in PK commonly have clinical implications. Gabapentin, levetiracetam and tiagabine do not induce or inhibit hepatic metabolism enzymes. Felbamate demonstrated an inducing effect on CYP 3A4 isoenzyme, and inhibition effect on CYP 2C19 and on β-oxidation of valproic acid. Lamotrigine induces its own metabolism, and some reports imply a decrease of valproic acid levels during concomitant treatment with lamotrigine. Oxcarbazepine induces CYP 3A4, 3A5, and uridine diphosphate glucuronyl transfereases (UGT), and inhibits the metabolism of phenytoin via CYP 2C19 isoenzyme. Similar induction and inhibition characteristics are attributed to topiramate, while some studies indicate that zonisamide may have inhibition potential on phenytoin metabolism.

In general, novel AEDs have linear PK, low plasma protein binding, and renal elimination, so their PK is more favorable in comparison with carbamazepine, phenobarbitone and valproic acid. This chapter gives a review of PK parameters of novel AEDs and its' variability based on age, comorbidities, concomitant therapy, and highlights the need of therapeutic drug monitoring.

1. Introduction

A choice of an antiepileptic drug (AED) is usually based upon the epileptic seizure type and syndrome, and drug characteristics. Novel AEDs increased the spectrum of epilepsy treatment (Stefan and Feuerstein, 2007). Among adverse effects, drug formulation, likelihood for drug interaction, pharmacokinetic (PK) profile should also be included in the choice of AED. PK characteristics of AEDs may be of valuable support in choosing the optimal therapeutic option for the individual patient.

AEDs are subdivided into older (first generation) drugs including carbamazepine, phenytoin, phenobarbitone, valproic acid; second generation – felbamate, gabapentin, lamotrigine, levetiracetam, oxcarbazepine, pregabalin, rufinamide, stiripentol, tiagabine, topiramate, vigabatrin, zonisamide; and third generation AEDs comprising eslicarbazepine acetate and lacosamide. When licensed, novel AEDs were generally used as adjunctive therapy, whereas nowadays they can be used in monotherapy as well (Patsalos and Bourgeois, 2010; Shorvon et al., 2009).

In comparison to first generation AEDs, novel AEDs have linear PK, low plasma protein binding, they are less prone to PK drug interactions, all of which makes their PK more predictable and easier to prescribe and to use in therapy. Although, these drugs belong to the same group their individual PK characteristics differ (Johannessen and Tomson, 2006; Splinter, 2005), and this chapter will outline the PK processes of new AEDs.

2. Pharmacokinetic Characteristics of Novel Antiepileptic Drugs

An overview of PK characteristics of each of the novel AEDs is presented through absorption, distribution and elimination parameters including metabolism and excretion, highlighting the factors contributing to the variability in PK. The summary of the typical values of AEDs' PK parameters is presented in the Table 1.

2.1. Eslicarbazepine Acetate

The field of indication for eslicarbazepine acetate is adjunctive therapy in adults with partial seizures with or without secondary generalization (Patsalos and Bourgeois, 2010).

The PK of eslicarbazepine is linear in the range 400-1200 mg both in healthy subjects and patients. Eslicarbazepine acetate is a pro-drug, rapidly and almost completely metabolized by hepatic esterases to eslicarbazepine which is further eliminated by kidneys as unchanged or in the glucuronide conjugate form. Minor active metabolites include oxcarbazepine and (R)-licarbazepine (Splinter, 2005). It has low binding to proteins with volume of distribution about 2.7 l/kg, so it is extensively cleared by hemodialysis. During therapy, its half-life is up to 24 h (Shorvon et al., 2009). Eslicarbazepine acetate metabolites are excreted primarily by the renal route, and their clearance is dependent on the renal function. In patients with a creatinine clearance less than 60 ml/min dosage adjustment may be necessary (Maia et al., 2008). On the other hand, the PK of eslicarbazepine acetate is not affected by moderate hepatic impairment, so patients with mild to moderate liver impairment do not require dosage adjustment of the drug (Almeida et al., 2008).

During concomitant therapy with topiramate or lamotrigine, no significant PK interaction was observed (Almeida et al., 2010; Nunes et al., 2010). However, an 18% decrease in exposure to topiramate was observed, most likely due to the reduced bioavailability of topiramate (Nunes et al., 2010). No dosage adjustments appear to be required routinely in either drug when the drugs are co-administered as well as when eslicarbazepine is combined with valproic acid, gabapentin, clobazam, or levetiracetam. In patients treated with inducing AEDs such as carbamazepine, phenobarbiton and phenytoin, eslicarbazepine elimination was found to be increased (Shorvon et al., 2009).

2.2. Felbamate

Primary indication for felbamate is mono- or adjunctive treatment of partial-onset seizures with or without secondary generalization in adults, and add-on therapy associated with Lennox-Gastaut syndrome in children (Patsalos and Bourgeois, 2010).

Felbamate is almost completely absorbed after *per os* administration, with high bioavailability (over 90%), and peak levels after 2-6 h of intake. Absorption of the drug is not affected by food. Approximately 20-25% of the drug is bound to albumin, and the apparent volume of distribution is estimated at about 0.8 l/kg (Shorvon et al., 2009).

Felbamate is equally eliminated unchanged in urine and metabolized in the liver via hydroxylation (through CYP 3A4, 2E1) followed by conjugation. About 15% is present as parahydroxyfelbamate, hydroxyfelbamate, and felbamate monocarbamate, none of which have significant anticonvulsant activity. Its half-life approximates 20 h, and multiple dosing does not appear to alter the elimination half-life.

Potent drug inductors of CYP 450 isoenzymes (e.g. carbamazepine, phenobarbitone, rifampicin) can increase its metabolism up to 40%, while valproic acid increases serum felbamate levels for up to 20% (Patsalos et al., 2008). On the other hand, felbamate demonstrated an inducing effect on the CYP 3A4 isoenzyme, and an inhibition effect on CYP 2C19 and on β-oxidation of valproic acid (Perucca, 2005; Shorvon et al., 2009). Clearance of felbamate may be higher in children, while in elderly there may be a minor decrease. In patients with decreased renal function, increase of a half-life depends on the level of impairment (Stefan and Feuerstein, 2007).

2.3. Gabapentin

This AED is indicated as adjunctive or monotherapy of partial or secondary generalized seizures (Patsalos and Bourgeois, 2010).

Gabapentin is rapidly absorbed from the gastrointestinal tract via active L-amino acid transport system reaching maximal drug levels 2-3 h after a single dose. Its bioavailability ranges from 40 to 60%. Marked nonlinear absorption is due to saturable L-amino acid transport system (Gidal et al., 1998) at doses higher than 4800 mg/day (Berry et al., 2003). Food does not influence its absorption. On the contrary, certain antacids (such as aluminum hydroxide, magnesium hydroxide) can decrease its bioavailability by up to one quarter, thus in order to avoid this interaction, these medications should be taken within 2 hours of each other (Shorvon et al., 2009). It is minimally or not bound to plasma proteins whatsoever, and is secreted into saliva and concentrations are similar to the unbound levels seen in plasma. Apparent volume of distribution is around 1 l/kg (Shorvon et al., 2009; Splinter, 2005).

Gabapentin undergoes, almost completely, renal elimination. Hence, patient's renal function has to be monitored. Its half-life is approximately 6 h, leading to dosing three times per day. In patients with decreased renal function, it is vital to adjust dose according to creatinine clearance. As a result of decreasing renal function by age, special care is needed when a drug is given to elderly patients. If the patient undergoes hemodialysis, close monitoring is required since the drug can be removed from the body so patients may require supplemental doses (Wong et al., 1995). Due to renal elimination, gabapentin is less likely to exhibit clinically important drug-drug interactions. However, cimetidine might decrease its renal clearance and increase gabapentin plasma levels (Shorvon et al., 2009).

2.4. Lacosamide

Lacosamide is used as adjunctive therapy of partial-onset seizures with or without secondary generalization in adults with epilepsy (Patsalos and Bourgeois, 2010).

The drug is reaching peak levels after 0.5-4 h of administration, and its bioavailability is almost complete. Food does not influence its absorption. It shows low protein binding with volume of distribution 0.5-0.8 l/kg (Shorvon et al., 2009).

Lacosamide is partially eliminated by excretion in unchanged form in the urine (40% of the administered dose), and partly by metabolism (primarily O-demethylation) followed by excretion. The drug is metabolized to inactive form via the CYP 2C9 isoenzyme. The influence of CYP 2C9 isoenzyme genetic polymorphism on plasma lacosamide concentrations is not fully elucidated (Beyreuther et al., 2007; Doty et al., 2007; Shorvon et al., 2009). Half-life is practically 12 h. Mild to moderate renal impairment results in increased lacosamide levels, so dosage reduction may be necessary in some patients, while in severe renal impairment (creatinine clearance below 30 mL/min) dosage regimens have to be reconsidered. Because lacosamide can be removed by hemodialysis, patients on hemodialysis may require supplemental doses of the drug. In the population of patients with decreased liver function, lower doses may be required. PK studies suggest that enzyme-inducing AEDs reduce serum lacosamide levels by about 25% (Doty et al., 2007; Stefan and Feuerstein, 2007).

Table 1. Pharmacokinetic characteristics of novel antiepileptic drugs (Patsalos and Bourgeois, 2010)

ANTIEPILEPTIC DRUG	F [%]	t_{max} [h]	PB [%]	Vd [l/kg]	Elimination	CL	$t_{1/2}$ [h]
Eslicarbazepine acetate	> 80	1–4	30[a]	2.7[a]	hydrolysis + conjugation + renal excretion	55 ml/h/kg	13–20[a]
Felbamate	> 90	2–6	20–25	0.8	oxidation + renal excretion	20–40 ml/h/kg	11–25
Gabapentin	40–60	2–3	0–10	0.65–1.04	renal excretion	1.3–1.6 ml/min/kg	5–9
Lacosamide	100	0.5–4	<15	0.5–0.8	renal excretion + metabolism	no data	12–16
Lamotrigine	> 90	1–3	50–60	0.9–1.3	metabolism (conjugation with glucuronides)	0.5–1.15 ml/min/kg	15–35
Levetiracetam	95	1	0	0.5–0.7	hydrolysis + renal excretion	0.9–1.3 ml/min/kg	6–8
Oxcarbazepine[b]	90	3–6	40	0.7–0.8[b]	metabolism	40–50 ml/h/kg	7–12[b]
Pregabalin	90	1–2	0	0.5	renal excretion	0.7–1.0 ml/min/kg	5–7
Rufinamide	85	5–6	30	0.8 (at 3200 mg /day)	metabolism (hydrolysis)	90 ml/h/kg (45mg/kg)	6–12
Stiripentol	90	1–2	99	not known	metabolism (glucuronide conjugation and O-methylation)	dose-dependent	4.5–13 dose-dependent
Tiagabine	90	1–2	96	1.2	oxidation	2–3 ml/min/kg	5–9
Topiramate	80–95	2–4	13–17	0.6–1.0	oxidation + renal excretion	15–50 ml/h/kg	10–30
Vigabatrin	60–80	1–2	0	0.8	renal excretion	0.10–0.144 l/h/kg	4–7
Zonisamide	65	2–5	40–50	1.1–1.8	renal excretion + metabolism (CYP3A4, *N*-acetyltransferase and glucuronyl transferases)	10–20 ml/h/kg	50–70

[a] refers to eslicarbazepine.

[b] refers to metabolite 10-hydroxycarbazepine.

F-absolute bioavailability; t_{max}-time to reach maximal levels; PB-protein binding; CL-clearance; $t_{1/2}$-half-life.

2.5. Lamotrigine

When registered, lamotrigine was indicated as add-on therapy for partial seizures. Nowadays, its indication field has been expanded to monotherapy for partial seizures and for treatment of bipolar disorders (Patsalos and Bourgeois, 2010).

Lamotrigine is rapidly and completely absorbed from the gastrointestinal tract reaching maximal concentrations 1-3 h after administration. Around 50-60% of the drug is bound to proteins, and volume of distribution is 0.9-1.3 l/kg (Shorvon et al., 2009; Splinter, 2005).

It has been shown that LTG induces its own metabolism, leading to approximately 20% decrease in drug levels in two weeks period. The main route of elimination is uridine diphosphate glucuronosyl transferease (isoform UGT 1A4) dependent conjugation to inactive metabolites (90% of administered dose). The half-life of lamotrigine is 15-35 h. During concomitant treatment with drugs that can induce its metabolism (e.g. ethinyl estradiol, carbamazepine) it can be decreased to 8-20 h, whereas with inhibitors such as valproic acid lamotrigine's half-life can be extended up to 60 h (Biton, 2006). Comparable effects are observed in pediatric patients (Brzaković et al., 2000; 2002). Oral contraceptives can increase the clearance of lamotrigine. Moreover, an alteration of valproic acid levels during concomitant treatment with lamotrigine is not observed (Vučićević et al., 2009) even some reports imply a decrease of valproic concentrations (Johannessen and Patsalos, 2010).

However, lamotrigine is eliminated via renal route as well. Hence, in patients with decreased kidneys function, its half-life can be increased to 50 h. Because lamotrigine can be removed by hemodialysis, patients may need additional doses of the drug after dialysis. Lamotrigine is extensively metabolized, and consequently lower doses will be essential in patients with hepatic impairment. Due to its safety profile, it is extensively used in pregnant patients (Sabers and Tomson, 2009; Wegner et al., 2010). However, an up to 3 times higher clearance of the drug has been observed in pregnant patients, leading to lower lamotrigine levels, which indicates the need for higher doses of the drug in this patient population (Perucca, 2006). The drug is excreted into breast milk reaching 40-80% of maternal plasma levels. In concordance, lamotrigine plasma levels in breastfed infants are 25-50% of maternal plasma levels.

2.6. Levetiracetam

Levetiracetam is used as first-line and add-on therapy of partial-onset seizures. Adjunctive and, possibly, first-line therapy of generalized tonic–clonic and myoclonic seizures associated with idiopathic generalized epilepsies (Patsalos and Bourgeois, 2010).

Levetiracetam is rapidly and almost completely absorbed after *per os* administration. It has been showed that food makes absorption slightly slower without effect on extent of absorption, but it has no clinical relevance (Fay et al., 2005). Levetiracetam is not bound to plasma proteins, and its volume of distribution approaches the volume of total body water (Patsalos, 2004). Levetiracetam is also distributed in blood cells (Stefan and Feuerstein, 2007).

The elimination of an unchanged drug is almost completely by kidneys; either unchanged (66%) or as hydrolyzed inactive metabolite created in the blood by amidase(s)/esterase(s) (Benedetti et al., 2003; Patsalos, 2004). Average half-life of a drug in adults is 6-8 h.

Therefore, elimination of a drug is dependent on patient's renal function. Consequently, dosage adjustments might be necessary in patients with moderate to severe renal impairment, since half-life seems to be prolonged in these patients by 35-60%. In patients on hemodialysis supplemental doses of levetiracetam may be required since the drug may be removed by dialysis. Clinically important PK interactions between levetiracetam and other AEDs have not been identified, since its metabolism is independent of CYP 450 isoenzymes, and due to the fact that amidases/esterases, even when inducible, are less prone to induction than CYPs and UGT (Benedetti et al., 2003). However, pharmacodynamic interactions with carbamazepine and topiramate have been observed resulting in increased potential for adverse drug reactions (Patsalos, 2004). Overall, levetiracetam has a favorable PK profile, which makes its clinical use simple and straightforward. Serum concentrations of levetiracetam are significantly reduced in the third trimester of pregnancy due to increased clearance, but they are raised rapidly after delivery (Tomson et al., 2007; Westin et al., 2008), indicating the need for monitoring.

2.7. Oxcarbazepine

Oxcarbazepine, as a keto-derivate of carbamazepine, has similar antiepileptic efficacy and is effective both as monotherapy and as adjunctive therapy for all types of partial seizures with or without secondary generalization. Above all, it might be useful in patients who do not tolerate carbamazepine but respond to it (Patsalos and Bourgeois, 2010).

Oxcarbazepine is rapidly and completely absorbed after oral administration. It can be given with or without food since its oral bioavailability is not affected by food intake. The volume of distribution value indicates its distribution into total body water (Johannessen and Tomson, 2006).

It is metabolized through 10-keto reduction by cytosolic aldo-ketoreductase enzymes to active equipotent enantiomers of 10,11-dihydro-10-hydroxycarbamazepine (monohydroxycarbazepine, licarbazepine) (96%), which reaches peak concentrations in 3-6 h. Further, it is conjugated with UGT. Most of oxcarbazepine administered dose in urine is in the form of monohydroxycarbazepine glucuronide (51%) and unchanged monohydroxycarbazepine (28%), while only 1% accounts for unchanged oxcarbazepine (Dickinson et al., 1989). As oxcarbazepine is rapidly eliminated from plasma, its half-life is small (around 1.5 h), and has no practical meaning, whereas the half-life of active metabolite is around 9 h. Unlike carbamazepine, an autoinduction phenomenon is not a feature of oxcarbazepine metabolism (Stefan and Feuerstein, 2007). Both oxcarbazepine and monohydroxycarbazepine exhibit low protein binding.

Mild to moderate hepatic dysfunction did not alter the PK of oxcarbazepine or its active metabolite, but in severe liver impairment prolonged half-life can be expected. Oxcarbazepine induces CYP 3A4, 3A5, and UGT (but less than carbamazepine), and inhibits the metabolism of phenytoin via the CYP 2C19 isoenzyme. Therefore, it can decrease plasma levels of carbamazepine, lamotrigine, and topiramate, and increase plasma levels of phenobarbital and phenytoin up to 40% (Johannessen and Patsalos, 2010).

Carbamazepine, phenobarbital, phenytoin, and primidone can increase clearance of monohydroxycarbazepine due to the induction mechanism. Concomitant administration with lamotrigine has been associated with an increased risk of adverse reactions such as nausea, somnolence, dizziness, and headache due to increased levels of lamotrigine (Johannessen and Patsalos, 2010).

2.8. Pregabalin

Pregabalin was introduced as adjunctive therapy for the treatment of partial seizures with or without secondary generalization (Patsalos and Bourgeois, 2010).

After oral administration pregabalin is rapidly absorbed with absolute bioavailability over 90%. Being a leucine analog, pregabalin is transported both into the blood and to the brain by the system L-transport system (a sodium-independent transporter) as well as by additional sodium-dependent amino acid transporter systems. Food decreases the rate of pregabalin absorption, resulting in lower and delayed maximum levels by approximately 2.5 h, yet the extent of absorption is unaffected, indicating possibility of the drug to be administered without regard to meals (Bockbrader et al., 2010). It is not bound to plasma proteins.

Pregabalin is eliminated completely via the renal route (98%) with a clearance reaching the value of glomerular filtration rate (Bockbrader et al., 2010). Consequently, in patients with decreased renal function, reduced dose is required and it is cleared by hemodialysis (Randinitis et al., 2003). The half-life ranges from 5 to 7 h, so steady-state is reached in 1-2 days.

Since it is not bound to plasma proteins, and elimination is not metabolism-based, PK drug-drug interactions are considered unlikely with pregabalin (Bockbrader et al., 2011), and it might be an alternative to patients with impaired hepatic function (Stefan and Feuerstein, 2007).

2.9. Rufinamide

Rufinamide is approved as add-on therapy for Lennox-Gastaut syndrome in patients older than 4 years (Patsalos and Bourgeois, 2010; Wier et al., 2011).

Following oral administration around 85% of the dose is absorbed. However the extent of absorption is dose-dependent since the bioavailability decreases with increased doses, presumably as a result of its slow dissolution into gastrointestinal contents. The drug follows linear PK up to 1600 mg/day, whereas nonlinear PK was observed at higher doses due to reduced oral bioavailability (Wier et al., 2011). Food influences the absorption profile of the drug, leading to significant increase in maximum drug levels in comparison to absorption from an empty stomach (Perucca et al., 2008). Maximum plasma values are increased by 100%, whereas time reaching maximum values is shortened (6 hours versus 8 hours when fasted).

Rufinamide is extensively metabolized by carboxylesterase to inactive metabolite that is excreted in the urine (70%) or feces (9%), while around 4% of an administered dose is excreted unchanged by kidneys. The plasma half-life is 6-12 h. In children clearance values can be expected up to 50% higher. Although the dosing regimen does not need to be adjusted for patients with decreased renal function special concern is required in patients undergoing hemodialysis. In patients with hepatic impairment lower doses may be required (Perucca et al., 2008; Wier et al., 2011).

Well-known metabolic inducers can increase the metabolism of rufinamide, while valproic acid can decrease its clearance and consequently increase plasma levels. Conversely, rufinamide can decrease plasma levels of carbamazepine and lamotrigine, and increase levels of phenobarbital and phenytoin (Johannessen and Patsalos, 2010).

2.10. Stiripentol

Stiripentol is used with clobazam and valproate in adjunctive therapy of refractory generalized tonic-clonic seizures in patients with severe myoclonic epilepsy in infancy (Dravet's syndrome) whose seizures are not adequately controlled with clobazam and valproate (Patsalos and Bourgeois, 2010).

Stiripentol is rapidly absorbed from the gastrointestinal tract after *per os* administration. The absolute oral bioavailability is high. It is highly bound to proteins (99%). Stiripentol should be taken with food, except food and drinks containing caffeine, because it degrades rapidly in an acidic environment, such as in gastric contents in a fasting state (Johannessen and Tomson, 2006).

The drug undergoes metabolism in the liver by desmethylation and glucuronidation, resulting in at least 13 identified inactive metabolites. The drug reveals nonlinear PK (Michaelis-Menten kinetics) that can be observed in non-proportional rise of a drug levels with increased dose due to saturable enzyme system involved in metabolism (Levy et al., 1983; 1984). The half-life of stiripentol is in the range of 4.5-13 h, and it is increasing with increasing dose (Stefan and Feuerstein, 2007).

Stiripentol shows clinically significant interactions with other AEDs, mainly as a result of stiripentol's ability to potently inhibit the activity of CYP 1A2, 2C9, 2C19, 2D6, and 3A4. Therefore, stiripentol increases the concentration of carbamazepine, phenobarbiton, phenytoin, clobazam, and, to less extent, valproic acid (Levy et al., 1984). The stiripentol's effect on carbamazepine metabolism builds up gradually over 7-10 days, indicating the need to adjust dosage regimen of carbamazepine. Enzyme-inducing AEDs increase stiripentol clearance by 300% (Johannessen and Patsalos, 2010; Levy et al., 1984).

2.11. Tiagabine

Tiagabine is indicated as adjunctive therapy of partial seizures, with and without secondary generalization (Patsalos and Bourgeois, 2010).

Tiagabine is rapidly absorbed, with high percentage of a drug bound to proteins (> 90%). Food delays the time to peak concentration from a mean of 1 h to a mean of 2.6 h, without affecting the extent of drug absorbed. Although tiagabine is highly bound to proteins, it does not displace highly protein-bound drugs (e.g. phenytoin and valproic acid) from their binding sites (Patsalos et al., 2008; Shorvon et al., 2009).

It is considerably metabolized via CYP 3A4 isoenzyme to inactive metabolites, further excreted via bile. The half-life ranges from 5 to 9 h. Tiagabine did not show either induction or inhibition potential for CYP 450 enzymes. However, the risk of PK interactions is high, particularly with those drugs that inhibit/induce CYP 3A4. Therefore, concomitantly used carbamazepine, phenobarbitone, phenytoin will decrease the half-life of tiagabine

(Johannessen and Patsalos, 2010). In patients with mild to moderate hepatic failure, adverse effects should be closely monitored, and dosing regimens might need an adjustment, while in severe hepatic failure the drug should be avoided. Nevertheless, the drug has unrestricted use in patients with renal insufficiency (Johannessen and Tomson, 2006).

2.12. Topiramate

Primary indications of topiramate are adjunctive or monotherapy in partial and secondary generalized seizures, as well as Lennox-Gastaut syndrome and primary generalized tonic-clonic seizures (Patsalos and Bourgeois, 2010).

Topiramate shows linear PK. After oral administration, topiramate is rapidly absorbed with bioavailability of 80-95%. Food does not affect its absorption. Volume of distribution of the drug is around 0.6-1 l/kg (Shorvon et al., 2009).

Topiramate is excreted unchanged through the kidneys (40-50%), although a fraction of the oral dose is metabolized, mostly by the CYP microsomal enzymes. At least 12 inactive metabolites have been identified, formed by hydroxylation, hydrolysis, glucuronide or sulphate conjugation or cleavage of the sulphamate group (Caldwell et al., 2005; Splinter, 2005). Based on its half-life value, it is needed 4-5 days to reach steady-state.

Due to the topiramate elimination route, lower doses may be required in patients with renal failure. Due to low protein binding it is suspected that topiramate might be cleared during dialysis. After hemodialysis, an additional dose (approximately half of the daily dose, in addition to the full daily dose) of topiramate may be necessary, because topiramate is cleared from plasma during dialysis at a rate which is approximately 4-6 times higher than in patients with normal renal function (Shorvon et al., 2009). Moreover, in patients with hepatic failure lower doses may be required too.

There are data suggesting that enzyme inducers can increase its clearance, reducing topiramate half-life from 20-30 h to 12 h (Bialer et al., 2004). Topiramate can decrease the clearance of phenytoin, and increase the clearance of valproic acid. However, topiramate effect on valproic acid is most likely dose-dependent (Vučićević et al., 2009a; 2009b).

2.13. Vigabatrin

Vigabatrin is indicated as monotherapy of infantile spasms (West syndrome). It may be of great value as adjunctive therapy for partial and secondary generalized seizures refractory to other drugs (Patsalos and Bourgeois, 2010).

Vigabatrin is a racemate mixture of two enantiomers, but only S(+)-enantiomer has pharmacological activity. Vigabatrin has bioavailability from 60 to 80%, and peak levels are reached within 2 h of *per os* administration. Food does not influence its absorption. It is not bound to plasma proteins, and is widely distributed in the body.

The major route of elimination is renal. Therefore, renal clearance of vigabatrin is proportional to the creatinine clearance. Hence, special care should be addressed to patients with renal diseases and older patients. The half-life value is around 6 h and 1-2 days are needed for steady-state.

Overall, vigabatrin has low potential for drug-drug interactions (Johannessen and Patsalos, 2010). Nevertheless, it was showed that vigabatrin may reduce serum phenytoin levels by about 25% (Gatti et al., 1993).

2.14. Zonisamide

Adjunctive therapy of partial and secondarily generalized and a variety of primary generalized seizure types are primary indications for zonisamide (Kothare and Kaleyias, 2008; Patsalos and Bourgeois, 2010).

Zonisamide is rapidly absorbed from the gastrointestinal tract, and its bioavailability is around 65%. Food co-ingestion delays the rate of absorption (4-6 h), but does not decrease the extent of absorption. The percent of the drug bound to plasma proteins is around 40-50%. It distributes in the body with volume of distribution 1-2 l/kg. Moreover, it is extensively accumulated in erythrocytes showing low-capacity binding to these blood cells (Patsalos et al., 2008).

It is predominantly metabolized. Zonisamide undergoes acetylation to N-acetyl zonisamide, and reduction to 2-sulfamoylacetylphenol by CYP 3A4 which is subsequently glucuronidated. The half-life is approximately 50-70 h. Hence, drug inducers and inhibitors affect PK parameters of zonisamide elimination. To date, there have been no reports of zonisamide affecting the PK of other AEDs (Kothare and Kaleyias, 2008).

3. Therapeutic Drug Monitoring of Novel Antiepileptic Drugs

Therapeutic Drug Monitoring (TDM) is a concept of individualisation of therapy based on drug concentration data, and application of PK and pharmacodynamic (PD) principles. TDM relies on the assumption that drug concentrations in biological fluids correlate better with clinical effects compared to the dose administered. It is not only a process of measuring drug concentration levels in biological fluids, but putting them into service of an optimized individual pharmacotherapy with minimal adverse drug effects (Patsalos, 2008; Patsalos and Bourgeois, 2010).

The necessity of TDM may be justified by disease-related and drug-related reasons. If there is uncertainty regarding the identification of therapeutic response or adverse drug reactions, TDM may be reasonable. Epilepsy is characterized by seizures which occur intermittently and usually unexpectedly, since it is an episodic disease, it is hard to say if a patient is in a seizure-free period or the effect of the treatment is satisfactory, which makes the clinical effect monitoring difficult. Moreover, the long-term treatment duration poses a risk for development of potentially serious adverse events; therefore lowest effective doses are required. From this point of view, it may be argued that TDM may be of considerable value in the treatment of epilepsy (Patsalos et al., 2008).

If individual AEDs are considered, there are several pharmacological properties which should be considered prior to initiating TDM. Drugs which exhibit pronounced inter-individual or intra-individual variability in PK, due to pharmacogenetics, age-related reasons, a narrow therapeutic range or based on drug-drug interactions, may be good candidates for TDM. However, monitoring will be valuable only if there is an existing and well established correlation between the drug concentration and therapeutic and/or toxic effects (Harden, 2000). In terms of PK, it may be supposed that drugs which act *per se,* have, linear PK, an unbound fraction at the sampling site which is equal to the unbound fraction at the receptor site and no active metabolites, will have a greater probability for a good correlation between the concentration in the biological sample (usually plasma) and the effect. Optimal sampling is essential in TDM. Therefore, it is considered that trough AEDs level is optimal since it represents characteristics of elimination phase (via clearance or half-life), with possibility of obtaining peak concentration as well. However, the majority of novel AEDs drugs are secreted into saliva and salivary concentrations are similar to the unbound levels seen in plasma. Therefore, this biological fluid can be used as an alternative to blood for routine TDM (Tomson and Johannessen, 2000).

Based on the presented PK characteristics of second generation AEDs, drugs whose routine TDM can be justified are lamotrigine, oxcarbazepine, stiripentol, and zonisamide due to interindividual variability in metabolism that reflects on PK parameters of elimination, namely clearance and half-life. Taking into account that these parameters are the core of adjusting dosing regimen e.g. the rate of drug administration (which represents the ratio of dose and dosing interval), it makes the importance to determine the individual clearance value in specific patient reasonable (Johannessen and Tomson, 2006; Patsalos et al., 2008). For other AEDs routine TDM might be considered in patients with impaired function of organs involved in drug elimination, or as a tool to assess patients' adherence (Tomson and Johannessen, 2000).

Table 2. Usual therapeutic ranges for novel antiepileptic drugs

ANTIEPILEPTIC DRUG	THERAPEUTIC RANGE [mg/l]
Eslicarbazepine acetate[a]	not defined
Felbamate	30 – 60
Gabapentin	12 – 20
Lacosamide	5 – 10
Lamotrigine	3 – 14
Levetiracetam	12 – 46
Oxcarbazepine[b]	3 – 35
Pregabalin	2.8 – 8.3
Rufinamide	not defined
Stiripentol	4 – 22
Tiagabine	20 – 200[c]
Topiramate	5 – 20
Vigabatrin	0.8 – 36
Zonisamide	10 – 40

[a] refers to metabolite eslicarbazepine.
[b] refers to metabolite 10-hydroxycarbazepine.
[c] ng/ml.

Therapeutic ranges for these drugs are not clearly defined, however there are results on correlation of usual drug levels and optimal response indicating wider therapeutic ranges in comparison to older AEDs (Table 2). Even without clear therapeutic range, individual therapeutic window might be set up in accordance to patient's response to the therapy. These individual references can be used in case of future treatment failures (Patsalos et al., 2008; Perucca, 2000).

For older AEDs there is a well defined but narrow therapeutic range, reflecting steady-state concentration known to be associated with a high possibility of seizure control and low risk of toxicity (Tomson and Johannessen, 2000). It has been shown that TDM is beneficial for older AEDs (Vučićević et al., 2007; 2009), however strong evidence is lacking on the importance of TDM of novel AEDs. Routine TDM data might be useful in developing population PK models that can quantify PK variability, and serve as a tool in individualization of epilepsy treatment (Vučićević et al., 2005).

Conclusion

Novel antiepileptic drugs have more favorable pharmacokinetic characteristics compared to older antiepileptic drugs including linear pharmacokinetics, and a lower extent of binding to plasma proteins. Elimination is mainly renal or non-cytochrome P450 dependent, which makes them less eligible to interact with other drugs during concomitant treatment. Hence, they might serve as attractive alternatives to first-generation antiepileptics. Therapeutic ranges for these drugs are not clearly defined; however there are results on correlation of usual drug levels and optimal response indicating wider therapeutic ranges. As far as routine therapeutic drug monitoring is considered, it might be an advantage for drugs that exhibit wide interindividual and intraindividual variability, and these data may be used in developing population pharmacokinetic models that can help in optimization of therapy of epilepsy.

Acknowledgments

The authors prepared this chapter as a part of the project *Experimental and Clinical-Pharmacological Investigations of Mechanisms of Drug Action and Interactions in Nervous and Cardiovascular System* (No 175023) funded by Ministry of Science and Technological Development, Belgrade, Republic of Serbia.

References

Almeida, L.; Nunes, T.; Sicard, E.; Rocha, J.F.; Falcão, A.; Brunet. J.S.; Lefebvre, M. and Soares-da-Silva, P. (2010). Pharmacokinetic Interaction Study Between Eslicarbazepine Acetate and Lamotrigine in Healthy Subjects. *Acta Neurologica Scandinavica*, 121, 257-264.

Almeida, L.; Potgieter, J.H.; Maia, J.; Potgieter, M.A.; Mota, F. and Soares-da-Silva, P. (2008). Pharmacokinetics of Eslicarbazepine Acetate in Patients with Moderate Hepatic Impairment. *European Journal of Clinical Pharmacology*, 64, 267-273.

Benedetti, M.S.; Whomsley, R.; Nicolas, J.M.; Young. C. and Baltes, E. (2003). Pharmacokinetics and Metabolism of 14C-Levetiracetam, a New Antiepileptic Agent in Healthy Volunteers. *European Journal of Clinical Pharmacology*, 59, 621-630.

Berry, D.J.; Beran, R.G.; Plunkeft, M.J.; Clarke, L.A. and Hung, W.T. (2003). The Absorption of Gabapentin Following High Dose Escalation. *Seizure,* 12, 28-36.

Beyreuther, B.K.; Freitag, J.; Heers, C.; Krebsfanger, N.; Scharfenecker, U. and Stohr, T. (2007). Lacosamide: A Review of Preclinical Properties. *CNS Drug Reviews,* 13, 21–42.

Bialer, M.; Doose, D.R.; Murthy, B.; Curtin, C.; Wang, S.S.; Twyman, R.E. and Schwabe, S. (2004). Pharmacokinetic Interactions of Topiramate. *Clinical Pharmacokinetics,* 43, 763-780.

Biton, V. (2006). Pharmacokinetics, Toxicology and Safety of Lamotrigine in Epilepsy. *Expert Opinion on Drug Metabolism and Toxicology,* 2, 1009-1018.

Bockbrader, H.N.; Burger, P. and Knapp, L. (2011). Pregabalin Effect on Steady-State Pharmacokinetics of Carbamazepine, Lamotrigine, Phenobarbital, Phenytoin, Topiramate, Valproate, and Tiagabine. *Epilepsia*, 52, 405-409.

Bockbrader, H.N.; Radulovic, L.L.; Posvar, E.L.; Strand, J.C.; Alvey, C.W.; Busch, J.A.; Randinitis, E.J.; Corrigan, B.W.; Haig, G.M.; Boyd, R.A. and Wesche, D.L. (2010). Clinical Pharmacokinetics of Pregabalin in Healthy Volunteers. *The Journal of Clinical Pharmacology*, 50, 941-950.

Brzaković, B.; Pokrajac, M.; Martinović, Ž.J.; Veličković, R. and Miljković, B.R. (2000). Therapeutic Monitoring of Lamotrigine in Children with Epilepsy on Polytherapy. *Abstract Book of 20th European Symposium on Clinical Pharmacy*, 11-14 October 2000, Basel, Switzerland, 12-A.

Brzaković, B.; Pokrajac, M.; Martinović, Ž.J.; Veličković, R.; Miljković, B.R. and Varagić, V.M. (2002). Disposition of Lamotrigine in Children with Epilepsy Receiving Politherapy, *Archives of Pharmacy*, 52, 668-669.

Caldwell, G.W.; Wu, W.N.; Masucci, J.A.; Mckown, L.A.; Gauthier, D.; Jones, W.J.; Leo, G. C. and Maryanoff, B. E. (2005). Metabolism and Excretion of the Antiepileptic/Antimigraine Drug, Topiramate in Animals and Humans. *European Journal of Drug Metabolism and Pharmacokinetics,* 30, 151-164.

Dickinson, R.G.; Hooper, W.D.; Dunstan, P.R. and Eadie, M.J. (1989). First Dose and Steady-state Pharmacokinetics of Oxcarbazepine and its 10-Hydroxy Metabolite. *European Journal of Clinical Pharmacology,* 37, 69–74.

Doty, P.; Rudd, D.; Stoehr, T. and Thomas, D. (2007). Lacosamide. *Neurotherapeutics*, 4, 145–148.

Fay, M.A.; Sheth, R.D. and Gidal, B.E. (2005). Oral Absorption Kinetics of Levetiracetam: the Effect of Mixing with Food and Enteral Nutrition Formulas. *Clinical Therapeutics*, 27, 594-598.

Gatti, G.; Bartoli, A. and Marchiselli, R. (1993). Vigabatrin-Induced Decrease in Phenytoin Concentration does not involve a Change in Phenytoin Bioavailability. *British Journal of Clinical Pharmacology,* 36, 603-606.

Gidal, B.E.; DeCerce, J.; Bockbrader H.N.; Gonzalez, J.; Kruger, S.; Pitterle, M.E.; Rutecki, P. and Ramsay R.E. (1998). Gabapentin Bioavailability: Effect of Dose and Frequency of Administration in Adult Patients with Epilepsy. *Epilepsy Research*, 31, 91-99.

Harden, C.Y. (2000). Therapeutic Safety Monitoring: What to Look for and When to Look for It. *Epilepsia,* 41S, S37-S44.

Johannessen, L.C. and Patsalos, P.N. (2010). Drug Interactions Involving the New Second- and Third-Generation Antiepileptic Drugs. *Expert Review of Neurotherapeutics*, 10, 119-140.

Johannessen, S.I. and Tomson, T. (2006). Pharmacokinetic Variability of Newer Antiepileptic Drugs. When is Monitoring Needed? *Clinical Pharmacokinetics,* 45, 1061-1075.

Kothare, S.V. and Kaleyias, J. (2008). Zonisamide: Review of Pharmacology, Clinical Efficacy, Tolerability, and Safety. *Expert Opinion on Drug Metabolism and Toxicology*, 4, 493-506.

Levy, R.H.; Lin, H.S.; Blehaut, H.M. and Tor, J.A. (1983). Pharmacokinetics of Stiripentol in Normal Man: Evidence of Nonlinearity. *The Journal of Clinical Pharmacology*, 23, 523-533.

Levy, R.H.; Loiseau, P.; Guyot, M.; Blehaut, H.M.; Tor, J. and Moreland, T.A. (1984). Stiripentol Kinetics in Epilepsy: Nonlinearity and Interactions. *Clinical Pharmacology and Therapeutics,* 36, 661-669.

Maia, J.; Almeida, L.; Falcão, A.; Soares, E.; Mota, F.; Potgieter, M.A.; Potgieter, J.H. and Soares-da-Silva, P. (2008). Effect of Renal Impairment on the Pharmacokinetics of Eslicarbazepine Acetate. *International Journal of Clinical Pharmacology and Therapeutics*, 46, 119-130.

Nunes, T.; Sicard, E.; Almeida, L.; Falcão, A.; Rocha, J.F.; Brunet, J.S.; Lefebvre, M. and Soares-da-Silva, P. (2010). Pharmacokinetic Interaction Study between Eslicarbazepine Acetate and Topiramate in Healthy Subjects. *Current Medical Research and Opinion*, 26, 1355-1362.

Patsalos, P.N. and Bourgeois, B.F.D. *The Epilepsy Prescriber's Guide to Antiepileptic Drugs*. Cambridge: Cambridge University Press; 2010.

Patsalos, P.N. (2004). Clinical Pharmacokinetics of Levetiracetam. *Clinical Pharmacokinetics,* 43, 707-724.

Patsalos, P.N.; Berry, D.J.; Bourgeois, F.D., Cloyd J.C.; Glauser, T.A.; Johannessen, S.I.; Leppik, I.E.; Tomson, T. and Perucca, E. (2008). Antiepileptic Drugs – Best Practice Guidelines for Therapeutic Drug Monitoring: A Position Paper by the Subcommission on Therapeutic Drug Monitoring, ILAE Commission on Therapeutic Strategies. *Epilepsia*, 49, 1239-1276.

Perucca, E. (2000). Is There a Role for Therapeutic Drug Monitoring of New Anticonvulsants? *Clinical Pharmacokinetics,* 38, 191-204.

Perucca, E. (2005). Clinically Relevant Drug Interactions with Antiepileptic Drugs. *British Journal of Clinical Pharmacology,* 61, 246-255.

Perucca, E. (2006). Clinical Pharmacokinetics of New-Generation Antiepileptic Drugs at the Extremes of Age. *Clinical Pharmacokinetics,* 45, 351-364.

Perucca, E.; Cloyd, J.; Critchley, D. and Fuseau, E. (2008). Rufinamide: Clinical Pharmacokinetics and Concentration-Response Relationships in Patients with Epilepsy. *Epilepsia*, 49, 1123-1141.

Randinitis, E.J.; Posvar, E.L.; Alvey, C.W.; Sedman, A.J.; Cook, J.A. and Bockbrader, H.N. (2003). Pharmacokinetics of Pregabalin in Subjects with Various Degrees of Renal Function. *The Journal of Clinical Pharmacology,* 43:277-283.

Sabers, A. and Tomson, T. (2009). Managing Antiepileptic Drugs during Pregnancy and Lactation. *Current Opinion in Neurology,* 22, 157-161.

Shorvon, S.; Perucca, E. and Engel, J editors. *The Treatment of Epilepsy*, 3rd edition, Oxford: Blackwell Publishing Ltd; 2009.

Splinter, M.Y. (2005). Pharmacokinetic Properties of New Antiepileptic Drugs. *Journal of Pharmacy Practice,* 18, 444-460.

Stefan, H. and Feuerstein, T.J. (2007). Novel Anticonvulsant Drugs. *Pharmacology and Therapeutics*, 113, 165-183.

Tomson, T. and Johannessen, S.I. (2000). Therapeutic Drug Monitoring of the New Antiepileptic Drugs. *European Journal of Clinical Pharmacology*, 55, 697-705.

Tomson, T.; Palm, R.; Källén, K.; Ben-Menachem, E.; Söderfeldt, B.; Danielsson, B.; Johansson, R.; Luef, G. and Ohman I. (2007). Pharmacokinetics of Levetiracetam during Pregnancy, Delivery, in the Neonatal Period, and Lactation. *Epilepsia*, 48, 1111-1116.

Vučićević, K.; Miljković, B.; Pokrajac, M. and Grabnar, I. (2009a). Effect of Topiramate on Valproic Acid Clearance in Adult Patients with Epilepsy: A Population Pharmacokinetic Study. *European Neuropsychopharmacology*, 19, S271.

Vučićević, K.; Miljković, B.; Pokrajac, M. and Petronijević, M. (2005). Population Pharmacokinetic Approach to Data Analysis. *Archives of Pharmacy*, 55, 483-496.

Vučićević, K.; Miljković, B.; Pokrajac, M.; Prostran, M.; Martinović, Ž. and Grabnar, I. (2009b). The Influence of Drug-Drug Interaction and Patients' Characteristics on Valproic Acid's Clearance in Adults with Epilepsy using Nonlinear Mixed Effects Modeling. *European Journal of Pharmaceutical Sciences*, 38, 512-518.

Vučićević, K.; Miljković, B.; Veličković, R.; Pokrajac, M.; Mrhar, A. and Grabnar, I. (2007). Population Pharmacokinetic Model of Carbamazepine Derived from Routine Therapeutic Drug Monitoring Data. *Therapeutic Drug Monitoring*, 29, 781-788.

Wegner, I.; Edelbroek, P.; Haan, G.J.; Lindhout, D.; Sander, J.W. (2010). Drug Monitoring of Lamotrigine and Carbamazepine Combination during Pregnancy, *Epilepsia,* 51, 2500-2502.

Westin, A.A.; Reimers, A.; Helde, G.; Nakken, K.O. and Brodtkorb, E. (2008). Serum Concentration/Dose Ratio of Levetiracetam before, during and dfter Pregnancy. *Seizure*, 17, 192-198.

Wier, H.A.; Cerna, A. and So, T.Y. (2011). Rufinamide for Pediatric Patients with Lennox-Gastaut Syndrome: A Comprehensive Overview. *Paediatric Drugs*, 13, 97-106.

Wong, M.O.; Eldon, M.A.; Keane, W.T.; Tirck, D.; Bockbrader H.N.; Underwood, B.A.; Sedman, A.J. and Halstenson, C.E. (1995). Disposition of Gabapentin in Anuric Subjects on Hemodialysis. *Journal of Clinical Pharmacology,* 35, 622-626.

In: Seizures and Anti-Epileptic Drugs
Editors: Willard Hosten and Aleph Burtsev
ISBN: 978-1-62100-255-0

Chapter V

Familial Cortical Myoclonic Tremor with Epilepsy

***Yang Lu*[1] *and Xuefeng Wang*[2*]**
[1] Department of Geriatrics
[2] Department of Neurology,
The First Affiliated Hospital of Chongqing Medical University,
Chongqing, China

Introduction

The association between tremor and epileptic seizures was firstly reported 36 years ago (Wakeno, 1975). In 1990, sporadic cases tremor with a cortical origin consisting of irregular, distal twitches of the extremities associated with seizures were named as cortical tremor (Ikeda et al., 1990). Subsequently, familial cases of cortical tremor, myoclonus and epileptic seizures, representing autosomal dominant inheritance were described under several names, such as familial adult myoclonic epilepsy (FAME), benign adult familial myoclonic epilepsy (BAFME), autosomal dominant cortical myoclonus and epilepsy (ADCME). The different acronyms for this syndrome are listed in the table 1. Recently, all of these syndromes were considered as one phenotype and proposed the term "familial cortical myoclonic tremor with epilepsy" (FCMTE). In briefly, FCMTE is an autosomal dominant disorder characterized by adult onset cortical tremor, myoclonus and seizures. The clinical features of FCMTE include involuntary rhythmic myoclonic movements (tremor) of the distal extremities, usually fingers movements, generalized tonic-clonic seizures (GTCS), and mental retardation. EEG shows generalized and focal spike and wave complexes. Somatosensory evoked potentials (SEP) indicated enlarged cortical components and enhanced long-loop reflex I (LLRI). Neuroimaging is usually normal although nonspecific abnormalities are sometimes reported in patients with mental retardation, such as mild enlargement of the subarachnoid spaces or of

[*] Corresponding to Prof. Xuefeng Wang, e-mail: xfyp@163.com.

the lateral ventricles. Antiepileptic drugs, including phenobarbital, valproic acid, benzodiazepines, are effective to this syndrome. Three loci have been identified on chromesome 8q23.3-q24.11, 2p11.1-q12.2 and 5p15.31-p15.

Pathophysiology

The pathophysiological and biochemical bases of this syndrome remain largely speculative to date. Cortical tremor has been observed in either genetic or symptomatic aetiology, including Angelman syndrome, ischaemic brain lesions involving sensorimotor cortex and surgical removal of frontal meningioma (Striano et al., 2005a). Hyperexcitability of sensorimotor cortex is demonstrated by electrophysiological studies; however, it is likely that enhanced excitability and deficits in inhibitory mechanisms may widespread more diffusely to cerebral cortex, as suggested by increased VEP amplitude and abnormal response to photic stimulation. Furthermore, a high propensity for intra-hemispheric and inter-hemispheric transcallosal spread has been suggested (Guerrini et al., 2001). However, whether the excessive excitability is due to the enhanced intrinsic rhythmic activity of cortical generators or to the abnormal reciprocal interactions with subcortical structures is still controversial.

This syndrome are related to cortical hyperexcitability of primary motor cortex, primary sensory cortex, or both, which are thought to be the result of decreased cortical inhibition by cerebello-thalamo-cortical projections possibly due to a changed γ-aminobutyric acid receptor function (van Rootselaar et al., 2005; Striano et al., 2005b). Cortical neurons are driven by a subcortical generator, or, alternatively, rhythmic motor cortex excitation can originate from rhythmic generators within the cortex. Brain MRI is usually normal except for some degree of generalized atrophy or a mild cerebellar atrophy. Postmortem examination showed a patchy atrophy of cerebellar cortex and a normal sensorimotor cortex in patients with cortical myoclonus. Visuospatial impairment has been reported in FCMTE family, this suggests an involvement of the ‘‘ventral pathway’’ related to a temporal lobe dysfunction (Suppa et al., 2009).

Table 1. Different acronyms of familial cortical myoclonic tremor syndromes with epilepsy (adapted from van Rootselaar et al. 2005)

Abbreviation	Full name
ADCME	Autosomal dominant cortical myoclonus and epilepsy
BAFME	Benign adult familial myoclonic epilepsy
Crt Tr	Cortical tremor
FAME	Familial adult myoclonic epilepsy
FCMT	Familial cortical myoclonic tremor
FCTE	Familial cortical tremor with epilepsy
FEME	Familial essential myoclonus and epilepsy
FMEA	Familial benign myoclonus epilepsy of adult onset
HTE	Heredofamilial tremor and epilepsy

In addition, the possible role of cerebellum has been suggested by neuropathological studies. The postmortem neuropathology in FCMTE patients showed cerebellar Purkinje cell degeneration and a normal sensorimotor cortex (van Rootselaar et al., 2004; 2007). Similar neuropathological changes have been found in other patients (Jay et al., 1991; Bhatia et al., 1995; Hayashi et al., 2001). The brain had no true atrophy. Macroscopically, no abnormalities were seen, brain stem and cerebellum weight was normal. Microscopy showed a few senile plaques in the frontal cortex and gyrus cinguli, temporal and parietal areas with a sporadic senile plaque. The motor cortex was normal. Some gliosis was seen in the claustrum. No abnormalities in substantia nigra, thalamus, subthalamus, hippocampus, pons and medulla oblongata was found. The cerebellar cortex and vermis revealed severe and diffuse loss of Purkinje cells and some Bergmann gliosis. Remaining Purkinje cells had an abnormal morphology including a stellate configuration with a poorly developed dendritic tree, short perisomatic dendrites and torpedoes, hyperchromatic cell nuclei, and sometimes two nuclei. Heterotopic Purkinje cells were found in the molecular layer. Empty basket cells were observed. A small hypoxic area was identified near the dentate nucleus with reactive gliosis. The pathological changes have suggested that cerebellar dysfunction involves in FCMTE. It is possible that loss of inhibitory cerebellar influence on motor cortical function may play an important rule in the genesis of myoclonus. Cortical hyperexcitability is possibly due to deficient cerebellar Purkinje cell inhibition via the cerebello-thalamo-cortical loop, or from a common mechanism as a channelopathy with secondary Purkinje cell degeneration (van Rootselaar et al., 2007).

Genetics

Genetic studies have identified three loci of FCMTE, including chromosome 8q23.3-q24.11 (FAME1/FCMTE1) (Mikami et al., 1999; Plaster et al., 1999), chromosome 2p11.1-q12.2 (FAME2/FCMTE3) (Guerrini et al., 2001; de Falco et al., 2003; Saint-Martin et al., 2008)., and 5p15.31-p152 (FAME3/FCMTE3) (Depienne et al., 2010). However, no corresponding gene has been found for this disease to date.

In 1991, linkage analysis showed that the first locus of FCMTE was assigned to the distal portion of 8q in a large Japanese kindred with benign adult familial myoclonic epilepsy (Mikami et al., 1999). A maximum 2-point LOD score of 4.31 with D8S555 was obtained, the maximum multipoint LOD score was 5.42 for the interval between D8S555 and D8S1779. The cytogenetic localization of 8q23.3-q24.11 was identified. This locus was proved in other 4 reported Japanese kindreds with familial adult myoclonic epilepsy (Plaster et al. 1999). They defined the FAME locus as a 4.6-cM region on chromosome 8q24 with a maximum LOD score of 4.86 flanked by markers D8S514 and D8S1804. Furthermore, the locus for benign adult familial myoclonic epilepsy is distinct from 3 other epilepsy-related loci on 8q: familial febrile convulsions-1 on 8q13-q21; KCNQ3 on 8q24; and childhood absence epilepsy on 8q24. (Mikami et al. 1999)

In 2001, genome-wide linkage analysis of the affected family with ADCME reported by localizing the suspect gene to the centromeric region of chromosome 2 with a maximum multipoint LOD score of 3.74 at marker D2S2175 (Guerrini et al., 2001), and this locus was mapped at chromosome 2p11.1-q12.2 with a maximum LOD score of 3.32 in 2 Italian families (de Falco et al. 2003). Moreover, this locus has been proved in other families (Labauge et al., 2002; Saint-Martin et al., 2008; Madia et al., 2008), and haplotype analysis identified a15-Mb region segregating. Sequence analysis of several candidate genes in that region did not identify pathogenic mutations.

In 2010, the third locus of FCMTE was identified in a large French family (Depienne et al., 2010). The genome-wide analysis found a single region on 5p15.31-p15 with a multipoint LOD score of 3.66. Further genotyping of all family members confirmed that the region spans 9.31 Mb between D5S580 and D5S2096. Two-point LOD scores of 6.3 for D5S486. The candidate genes of this region contain at least 23 genes, most of which are expressed in the brain. Sequencing of 2 candidate genes (*SEMA5A* and *CTNND2*) failed to detect any point mutation.

Clinical Manifestation

Tremor

Cortical tremor or myoclonic tremor in FCMTE is characterized by fast, small-amplitude myoclonic rhythmic jerks, which mainly involve in fingers and hands, and tremor may extend to lower limbs and occasionally to head or trunk. This tremor may be present at rest, and mainly provokes by posture and action, sometimes the tremor aggravates by emotional stress or lack of sleep. The severity of tremor varies between and within pedigrees from no functional impairment, more often moderate impairment (for example during writing), or occasionally to a severe functional impairment for all precise hand movements or for walking as it was described in some members of European families. Usually tremor is the first symptom that appears at the initiation of the disorder. Age of onset ranged from 10 to 60 years with an average around 35 years (van Rootselaar et al., 2005; Regragui et al., 2006).

Myoclonus

In addition to cortical tremor, most patients present distal segmental, arrhythmic, erratic myoclonic jerks at upper limbs, which are enhanced by posture and action. Onset of myoclonus is difficult to establish but usually it starts at around the same age as cortical tremor (Striano et al., 2009).

Epilepsy

Epileptic seizure commonly appears secondly after tremor; only 16% of cases represent seizures as the first symptom. In 82% of cases, it is a generalized tonic–clonic seizure. In addition, absences or myoclonic seizures or complex partial seizures were described in Italian pedigrees. Seizure frequency varied within and between pedigrees but most often there is a good response to antiepileptic drugs and a good spontaneous outcome. However our literature review indicates that, compared with Japanese patients, some European patients had more frequent seizures, requiring an association of antiepileptic drugs and with a worse outcome.

Additional Clinical Symptoms

Mental retardation was associated with myoclonic tremor and epilepsy in the two Italian families (Elia et al., 1998; Guerrini et al., 2001). Mild cognitive impairment (short-term memory, attention deficit) was reported in six Dutch patients and could not be only explained by the use of antiepileptic drugs. Night blindness was reported in a Japanese family (Manabe Y et al., 2002) and a migraine in a Turkish family (Saka et al., 2000).

Electrophysiology

Electrophysiological study is essential to confirm the cortical origin of myoclonus. However, some of these electrophysiological features can be masked by antiepileptic treatments. It is therefore recommended to stop antiepileptic drugs before performing the electrophysiological evaluation (Regragui et al., 2006).

(1) Polymyographic Recordings

Surface EMG helps differentiate tremor and myoclonus. It shows relatively rhythmic irregular 8–13 Hz bursts of short duration (50 ms), weak amplitude mainly in the distal muscles of the upper limbs. The EMG pattern is consistent with irregular rhythmic myoclonic jerks triggered by posture or action but sometimes present at rest.

(2) EEG

Spikes or poly-spike wave complexes were reported in most of patients with epilepsy and half of the affected relatives without epilepsy. Photoparoxysmal response was also reported in some affected patients..

(3) SEPs

A giant cortical response (P25–N33 amplitude larger than 8.5–15 μV) after stimulation of the median nerve at the wrist was reported in 84% of cases [13]. Cortical SEPs recorded in six patients from the Spanish family described (Labauge et al. 2002)

(4) Long-latency Reflex or C Reflex

A long-latency (40 ms) C reflex response, evoked at rest by stimulation of the median nerve in the Abductor Pollicis Brevis muscle was observed in most patients. It is probably the more reliable electrophysiological criterion to confirm the cortical origin of the myoclonus.

(5) Jerk-locked back-averaging EEG

The presence of a pre-movement cortical spike time-locked to the myoclonus and recorded on the sensorimotor cortex contralateral to the recorded myoclonus was reported in 60% of cases (van Rootselaar et al., 2005; Regragui et al., 2006).

Neuroradiology

MRI study is usually normal even if minor, nonspecific abnormalities (e.g., mild enlargement of the subarachnoid spaces of the lateral ventricles) are sometimes reported. MRI spectroscopy study demonstrated elevated choline/creatine ratio in the cerebellum cortex of patients with BAFME, compared with healthy controls. Other innovative neuroimaging approaches, such as MRI volumetry, voxelbased morphometry, positron emission tomography, single photon emission computed tomography, may also be an adjunctive tool supporting the diagnosis (Striano et al., 2009).

Reported Families with FCMTE

In 1990, it was firstly reported 2 Japanese patients with a disorder characterized by adult-onset of non-progressive postural and action finger tremor, seizures. A family history of the condition was found either. EMG showed that the tremor was associated with a relatively rhythmic discharge at a rate of 9 Hz, resembling essential tremor. However, electrophysiologic studies revealed giant somatosensory evoked potentials (SEPs) with enhanced long-loop C-reflexes, and premovement cortical spikes by the jerk-locked averaging method, all these features suggested such tremors originated from cortex, and the involuntary movements or cortical tremors were a form of cortical reflex myoclonus. The patients responded to anticonvulsants, such as clonazepam, valproate, and primidone, rather than beta-blockers. (Ikeda et al., 1990)

In 1996, Kuwano et al. (1996) presented pedigrees of 5 Japanese kindreds with benign adult familial myoclonic epilepsy (BAFME) inherited in a clear autosomal dominant pattern. Affected patients had myoclonus or epilepsy and abnormal EEG findings, particularly photosensitivity in the EEG. The age of onset of the disorder was between 18 and 50 years (Kuwano et al., 1996).

In 1997, 6 patients from 3 families with autosomal dominant familial cortical myoclonic tremor were described (Terada et al., 1997). The manifestation of patients included rhythmic involuntary movements in their upper and lower extremities which were induced particularly by posture and action. All patients had adult onset (mean 37 years). Three patients had rare seizures of loss of consciousness. EEG showed generalized spike and wave complexes, and photosensitivity in 4 patients was recorded. Electrophysiologic studies reflected cortical reflex myoclonus.

Other 3 families with adult-onset myoclonic epilepsy were also reported in 1997. Onset of the myoclonus was between 30 and 50 years, followed by rare generalized tonic-clonic seizures (GTCS). The disorder appeared to be autosomal dominant inheritance and was non-progressive. Electrophysiologic analysis showed polyspikes on EEG, giant wave SEPs, enhanced C-reflexes, and a preceding wave on JLA, which suggested the myoclonus originated in the cerebral cortex (Okino 1997).

In 1998, Elia et al. described a European family with cortical tremor, epilepsy, and mental retardation inherited in an autosomal dominant pattern. All 4 living patients examined had non-progressive postural and action 6- to 8-Hz tremor of the fingers, which was aggravated by emotional stress. Three patients had GTCS, which were well-controlled with treatment (phenobarbital and/or benzodiazepines). The 2 youngest patients in a later generation had a more severe phenotype, with earlier onset of symptoms (age 5 years) and moderate mental retardation. All patients showed diffuse spike-wave complexes on EEG and a photoparoxysmal response. Giant SEPs, enhanced C-reflex, and premyoclonus spike on JLA occurred in all patients (Elia M et al., 1998).

In 2001, a large Italian family in which 11 individuals (8 living) over 5 generations were described with an autosomal dominant pattern (Guerrini et al., 2001). The characterization included distal myoclonus and seizures. All affected members had onset in adulthood (mean 25 years) of distal, rhythmic involuntary movements resembling tremors, and infrequent GTCS. Three patients also had intractable complex focal seizures, which were often followed by secondary generalization. EEG showed focal frontotemporal as well as generalized interictal abnormalities. Detailed neurophysiologic studies revealed giant somatosensory evoked potentials (SEPs), enhanced long-loop C-reflexes, and premovement cortical spikes by the jerk-locked averaging method (JLA). The finding suggested a cortical origin. The affected patients had diffuse cortical hyperexcitability and a high propensity for intra- and interhemispheric cortical spread. Neuropsychologic testing suggested that 3 members had mild to moderate mental retardation and several patients had low or low-normal intellectual functioning.

In 2002, Labauge et al reported a 4-generation European family with clinical findings of FAME segregating in an autosomal dominant inheritance. Ten living and 3 deceased members had onset of symptoms after age 30 and a history of myoclonic movements of the extremities, and 8 of 13 also had GTCSs. Five patients underwent electrophysiologic examination with findings consistent with the diagnosis of FAME. Dementia and cerebellar ataxia were absent.

In 2002, Van Rootselaar et al also reported a large Dutch family in which 13 members had cortical tremor and epilepsy with an autosomal dominant inheritance. Tremulous movements resembling essential tremor were first noticed between ages 12 and 45 years. Generalized tonic-clonic seizures and myoclonic seizures began between 20 and 63 years, usually after the tremor. Symptom progression and severity varied from mild to severe. Several affected family members had cognitive impairment, such as short-term memory loss and attention deficits. No pyramidal or cerebellar signs were found, and electrophysiologic studies suggested cortical hyper-excitability. Certain anti-epileptic medications were useful. Cerebellar degeneration with neuronal loss, loss of Purkinje cell dendritic trees and gliosis were further detected in postmortem examination of an affected woman from the family, This patient had progressive irregular trembling of the limbs since age 35, myoclonic and generalized tonic-clonic seizures since age 38, and. memory deficits, hyperactive reflexes, action tremor, myoclonus, and intractable seizures at age of 68 years (van Rootselaar et al., 2002; 2004).

In 2003, 2 Italian families with nonprogressive autosomal dominant BAFME were reported (de Falco et al., 2003). Cortical tremor was the presenting symptom in all affected patients, appearing at age 11 to 40 years (mean in the twenties). Most patients had infrequent seizures, and electrophysiologic studies were consistent with cortical origin. Treatment with adrenergic beta-blockers was ineffective, but anticonvulsants such as clonazepam and valproate were effective.

In 2005, a BAFME Chinese family was reported, composing of 116 individuals in seven generations. 14 members were affected with distal, rhythmic myoclonus, resembling tremors at upper limbs, enhanced by fatigue and anger. Five members had infrequent generalized tonic–clonic seizures, and additional 13 members were affected with both myoclonus and rare generalized tonic–clonic epilepsy. The average age of onset was 34 years. Most patients experienced the first attack at the second or third decade, except for in the youngest generation at earlier (5-14 years). EEG recorded moderate to high amplitude polyspike wave or sharp and slow complex wave with bilateral frontal or occipital predominance. The course of the pedigree showed no progression. No ataxia and dementia were found in any patients (Deng et al., 2005).

In 2006, a large Italian family with autosomal dominant early-onset cortical myoclonus, photic-induced myoclonus and epilepsy over 5 generations was discovered (Gardella et al., 2006). Rhythmic CM of childhood onset was present in all 16 affected individuals (onset ranging from 3 to 12 years), photic-induced myoclonic jerks in 7, and epileptic seizures in 6 (onset ranging from 23 to 34 years). Five children of the fifth generation manifested also episodes of arousal with generalized tremor in early infancy ("tremulous arousals"). Jerk-locked back-averaging of rhythmic cortical myoclonus of six affected individuals, documented a premyoclonic EEG correlate.

In 2007, Carr et al reported 2 large families from South Africa with generalized tonic-clonic seizures and myoclonus. The mean age at onset was 20 years (range 13 to 31). Myoclonus predominantly affected the trunk and upper limbs but was also observed in the lower limbs. Hand tremor became apparent on posture holding. Additional features included nystagmus, abnormal pursuit, dysarthria, hyperreflexia, cerebellar ataxia, and cerebellar atrophy. A number of patients also had progressive cognitive impairment, resulting in dementia. EEG studies were abnormal in the majority of patients, with polyspike and wave activity and/or clear epileptogenic activity. Postmortem examination of 1 patient showed cerebellar atrophy and cerebellar neuronal loss. Several patients died in their thirties and forties. The families were of mixed ancestry, predominantly resulting from intermarriage between the original inhabitants of the area, the Khoi-San, and early settlers of European origin. The phenotype was earlier onset, more severe and also progressive compared to typical FAME1 and FAME2 (Carr et al., 2007).

In 2009, a three-generation Italy family with FCMTE was reported. Affected members of the family had tremor, myoclonus, epilepsy, and cognitive impairment. Epilepsy was mainly characterized by generalized tonic–clonic seizures or complex partial seizures followed by generalization. The neuropsychological assessment demonstrated that all affected members had a visuospatial impairment that was more evident in patients with low IQ scores. EEG recorded generalized cortical hyperexcitability and the lack of a premovement cortical potential in the back-averaging recording. TMS in the clinically affected members showed reduced MTh, CSP and SICI, suggesting hyperexcitability of primary motor cortex. The SAI and LAI tests were normal, indicating normal sensorimotor integration in this family (Suppa et al., 2009).

In 2009, Magnin et al described a five generations of French FCMTE with 76 family members. Mean age at onset in the 17 living patients was 28.8 years ranged from 24 to 41 years. All affected members had myoclonus/cortical tremor, and 65% of patients had generalized tonic-clonic seizures. Other clinical symptoms included photosensitivity in 94% of patients, partial seizures in 29% cases, sensitivity to starvation/exercise 35% of cases, vibration in 23% of cases, ophthalmic migraine 35% of cases and gait disorders in 59% of patients. The pattern of inheritance was consistent with autosomal-dominant inheritance, however, the FAME1 and FAME2 loci for FCMTE were excluded (Magnin et al., 2009).

In 2010, a large French family with FCMTE was described. 16 family members were affected, and the mean age at onset was 27.6 years (range 10–41 years). First symptoms were cortical myoclonus in 5 patients, seizures in 5 patients, and both at the same time in 6 patients. Two patients had only cortical myoclonus without seizures. Seizure types included generalized tonic-clonic seizures in 11 patients, and focal seizures in 3 patients. Focal seizures were characterized by visual hallucinations (colored flashes or geometric figures), pure transient loss of consciousness (<20 seconds), without automatism. Light and high contrast stimulation induced discomfort, worsened cortical myoclonus or triggered seizure. In addition, status epilepticus was observed in 2 patients. Seven patients aged older than 60 years (mean age 66, range 60–72) had severe myoclonus affecting both upper and lower limbs. Mental retardation and cognitive impairment were not observed.

In personal practice, a pedigree of FCMTE was identified in four successive Chinese Han generation (shown in Figure). The family comprised a total of 60 family members including 16 affected individuals with an autosomal dominant mode of inheritance. Most affected members had onset in adulthood (mean 35.1 years). Only one affected member (V7) had tremor at his age of 15 years old without seizure. All 13 affected living members had tremors. Seizures occurred in 9 living patients, including 3 patients with complex focal seizures, followed by secondary generalized seizures, and 6 patients with GTCSs. The frequency of seizure was ranged from 1 per month to 2 per lifetime. Typical case (III5): a 64-year-old female. She had her first seizure at the age of 40 years old. The manifestation included focal seizure with secondary generalized tonic-clonic seizure and tremor. The aura was uncomfortable feeling of fear. The frequency of seizure was once per month. CT scan of brain showed cerebral atrophy. EEG showed spike-wave discharges. Phenytoin was prescribed for controlling seizures, no seizure occurred during 2 years follow-up.

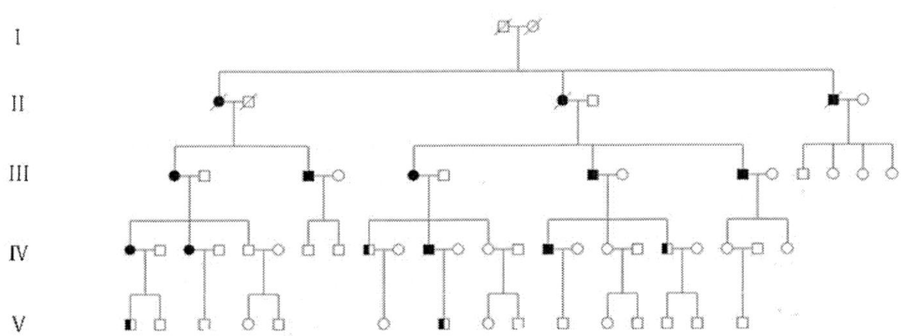

Circles and squares denote females and males, respectively. Affected individuals with tremulous finger movement and seizure are shown in black. Affected individuals with tremulous finger movement are shown in half-filled black Deceased family members are indicated by slashed symbols.

Summary

This syndrome is characterized by adult onset with nonprogressive course. Mean onset age is 37 years, ranged from 12 to 59 years, childhood onset has been reported. Tremor is often the first symptom: involuntary rhythmic myoclonic movements of the distal extremities, usually fingers; tremors characterized by 8 to 10-Hz discharges. Tremor may be elicited by movement or postural maintenance; tremor is aggravated by emotional stress. Patients have infrequent GTCS, myoclonus or intractable complex partial seizures, which were often followed by secondary generalization. In addition, mental retardation has been reported. EEG shows generalized and focal spike, polyspikes, spike-wave complexes and wave complexes, and photoparoxysmal response on EEG. Electrophysiologic analyses indicate a cortical origin, giant wave somatosensory evoked potentials, enhanced C-reflexes, and Jerk-locked premyoclonus spikes.

Diagnosis

The clinical diagnosis of FCMTE is based on the presence of adult onset, an irregular tremor-like myoclonic of the limbs, a (family) history of seizures, autosomal dominant inheritance, and a rather benign course. The finding of features of cortical reflex myoclonus strongly supports the diagnosis.

Clinical criteria include: 1) Familial autosomal dominant inheritance; 2) adult onset (between 20 and >70 yr). 3) distal predominance of involuntary, oscillatory, irregular, tremor-like myoclonic; 4) jerks in upper +/- lower limbs usually without involvement of trunk and head; 5) enhancement by outstretched posture and action, tiredness/sleep deprivation, caffeine, vibration, glucose deprivation, intense visual and/or auditory stimulation or contrast; 6) association with epilepsy; 7) no other neurological features, especially ataxia and cognitive impairment; 8) insidious course with slow or absent progression; 9) resistance to beta-blockers; 10) response to antiepileptic drugs (Bourdain et al., 2006).

Electrophysiological criteria include: 1) Brief electromyographic burst lasting less than 100 msec; 2) giant cortical components of SEPs; 3) enhanced long-loop C-reflex; 4) cortical spikes preceding myoclonic jerks at JLBA. Electrophysiological criteria are not required if they were found positive in another family member.

Differential Diagnosis

This disorder should be distinct from essential tremor and essential myoclonus, as well as from progressive myoclonic epilepsy and DRPLA (Terada et al., 1997).

Essential tremor (ET) is a progressive neurological condition that causes a rhythmic trembling of the arms, but the head, legs, trunk, voice, jaw, and facial muscles also may be involved. Aggravated by emotions, hunger, fatigue, and temperature extremes, the condition may cause a functional disability or even incapacitation. The onset of essential tremor is usually >50years, tremor may progress; no myoclonus and epileptic seizures exist. Tremor responds to β-blockers, and worsens by valproate (Bourdain et al., 2006). These features of essential tremor help the differential diagnosis from FCMTE. In addition, a coherence analysis suggests that cortical drive with centered around 17 Hz originated from the pre- or primary motor cortex leads to the fine distal tremulous movements in FCMTE. Corticomuscular and intermuscular coherence may also occur in ET with a frequency band centered around 6 Hz. Therefore, coherence analysis, in particular intermuscular coherence, may provide a sensitive tool for differentiating FCMTE from ET in the clinic (van Rootselaar et al., 2006).

Hereditary essential myoclonus, also named as myoclonic dystonia, is a genetically heterogeneous disorder characterized by myoclonic jerks affecting mostly proximal muscles. Dystonia is observed in most patients, but occasionally can be the only symptom of the disorder. Onset of the disorder is usually in the first or second decade. Symptoms often respond to alcohol, and patients can also have psychiatric abnormalities (Valente et al., 2003; Schule et al., 2004). In detail, myoclonus-dystonia is a movement disorder that typically affects the upper half of the body. Individuals with this condition experience quick, involuntary muscle jerking or twitching (myoclonus) that usually affects their arms, neck, and trunk. Less frequently, the legs are involved as well. More than half of affected individuals also develop dystonia, which affects a single part of the body, causing isolated problems such as a writer's cramp in the hand, or it may involve multiple areas of the body. Rarely, people with this condition have dystonia as their only symptom. The movement problems usually appear in childhood or early adolescence, and myoclonus is typically the initial symptom. Myoclonus may be triggered by movement or stimulation of the affected body area, stress, sudden noise, or caffeine. Myoclonus-dystonia is inherited in an autosomal dominant pattern, and mutations in the *SGCE* gene cause this disease.

Progressive myoclonic epilepsy is a rare epilepsy syndrome caused by a variety of genetic disorders, including Unverricht-Lundborg disease, myoclonus epilepsy and ragged red fibres, Lafora disease, neuronal ceroid lipofuscinoses, type I sialidosis, dentatorubropallidoluysian atrophy (DRPLA), the noninfantile neuronopathic form of Gaucher disease, and atypical inclusion body disease. It consists of both myoclonic seizures and tonic-clonic seizures together with progressive neurological decline. The myoclonus in PME is usually severe and is the prominent seizure type. Myoclonic seizures involve brief involuntary muscle twitching, and may become frequent enough to be disabling. Other symptoms can include uncontrollable sneezing, rapid blinking, and dwarfs. Neurological dysfunction includes difficulty coordinating muscle movements (ataxia) and a decline in cognitive ability (dementia). The initial effectiveness of anticonvulsant treatment diminishes as seizures become more frequent and neurological decline progresses.

Dentatorubral Pallidoluysian Atrophy (DRPLA) is an autosomal dominant condition, characterized by cerebellar ataxia, myoclonus, seizures, choreoathetosis and dementia. Mean age of onset 30 years (range first to seventh decade). Degeneration of the dentatorubral and pallidoluysian systems has been found in neuropathology. Molecular study indicates that this disorder is caused by trinucleotide repeat expansion (CAG)n in the DRPLA gene.

Treatment

Cortical tremor is not responsive to alcohol or beta-blockers, L-dopa/carbidopa. However, antiepileptic drugs (AEDs) are effective, especially phenobarbital, valproic acid, clonazepam. Other AEDs such as clobazam, phenytoin and carbamazepine have been reported to be effective for the severe epilepsy. Other antimyoclonic drugs, such as piracetam, levetiracetam and 5-OH-tryptophan seem to be less effective. Epilepsy has usually a benign course in patients taking antiepileptic therapy. However, complex partial seizures are drug-resistant (Striano et al., 2005).

It is well reported that antiepileptic drugs, such as benzodiazepines, valproate acid, primidone, carbamazepine, and lamotrigine seem to have the best efficacy to ameliorate the disability of patients (Bourdain et al., 2006). Topiramate 400 mg/day was not effective when given to the propositus (Patient III-7). Cortical and noncortical myoclonus can be treated successfully with levetiracetam. In general, valproate acid remains the first treatment option, as its efficacy upon seizures and cortical myoclonus is well known. Levetiracetam can be an alternative proposition if any contraindication or side effect limit valproate acid use, or in addition in case of partial efficacy of valproate acid upon the myoclonic tremor (Bourdain et al., 2006).

References

Bhatia KP, Brown P, Gregory R, Lennox GG, Manji H, Thompson PD, Ellison DW, Marsden CD. Progressive myoclonic ataxia associated with coelic disease. The myoclonus is of cortical origin, but the pathology is in the cerebellum. *Brain* 1995;118:1087-1093.

Bourdain F, Apartis, E, Trocello JM, Vidal JS, Masnou P, Vercueil L, Vidailhet M. Clinical analysis in familial cortical myoclonic tremor allows differential diagnosis with essential tremor. *Mov Disord* 2006; 21: 599–608.

Carr JA, van der Walt PE, Nakayama J, FuYH, Corfield V, Brink P, Ptacek L. FAME3: a novel form of progressive myoclonus and epilepsy. *Neurology* 2007; 68: 1382-1389.

de Falco FA, Striano P, de Falco A, Striano S, Santangelo R, Perretti A, Balbi P, Cecconi M, Zara F. Benign adult familial myoclonic epilepsy: genetic heterogeneity and allelism with ADCME. *Neurology* 2003; 60: 1381-1385.

Deng FY, Gong J, Zhang YC, Wang K, Xiao SM, Li YN, Lei SF, Chen XD, Xiao B, Deng HW. Absence of linkage to 8q23.3-q24.1 and 2p11.1-q12.2 in a new BAFME pedigree in China: indication of a third locus for BAFME. *Epilepsy Res* 2005; 65: 147-152.

Depienne C, Magnin E, Bouteille, D, Stevanin G, Saint-Martin C, Vidailhet M, Apartis E, Hirsch E, LeGuern E, Labauge P, Rumbach L. Familial cortical myoclonic tremor with epilepsy: the third locus (FCMTE3) maps to 5p. *Neurology* 2010; 74: 2000-2003.

Elia M, Musumeci SA, Ferri R, Scuderi C, Del Gracco S, Bottitta M, Michelucci R, Tassinari CA. Familial cortical tremor, epilepsy, and mental retardation: a distinct clinical entity? *Arch Neurol* 1998; 55: 1569-1573.

Gardella E, Tinuper P, Marini C, Guerrini R, Parrini E, Bisulli F, Liguori R, Montagna P, Lugaresi E. Autosomal dominant early-onset cortical myoclonus, photic-induced myoclonus, and epilepsy in a large pedigree. *Epilepsia.* 2006; 47(10): 1643-9.

Guerrini, R., Bonanni, P., Patrignani, A., Brown, P., Parmeggiani, L., Grosse, P., Brovedani, P., Moro, F., Aridon, P., Carrozzo, R., Casari, G. Autosomal dominant cortical myoclonus and epilepsy (ADCME) with complex partial and generalized seizures: a newly recognized epilepsy syndrome with linkage to chromosome 2p11.1-q12.2. *Brain* 2001; 124: 2459-2475.

Hayashi M, Endo K, Suzuki T et al. Benign adult familial myoclonic epilepsy: an autopsy case of homozygous affected individual. *Neuropathology* 2001; 21(Suppl. 21):106.

Ikeda, A., Kakigi, R., Funai, N., Neshige, R., Kuroda, Y., Shibasaki, H. Cortical tremor: a variant of cortical reflex myoclonus. *Neurology* 1990; 40: 1561-1565.

Jay V, Becker LE, Chan FW, Perri TL. Puppet-like syndrome of Angelman: a pathologic and neurochemical study. *Neurology* 1991; 41: 416-422.

Kuwano A, Takakubo F, Morimoto Y, Uyama E, Uchino M, Ando M, Yasuda T, Terao A, Hayayma T, Kobayashi R, Kondo I. Benign adult familial myoclonus epilepsy (BAFME): an autosomal dominant form not linked to the dentatorubral pallidoluysian atrophy (DRPLA) gene. *J Med Genet* 1996; 33: 80-81.

Labauge P, Amer LO, Simonetta-Moreau M, Attane F, Tannier C, Clanet M, Castelnovo G, An-Gourfinkel I, Agid Y, Brice A, Ducros A, LeGuern E. Absence of linkage to 8q24 in a European family with familial adult myoclonic epilepsy (FAME). *Neurology* 2002; 58: 941-944.

Magnin E, Vidailhet M, Depienne C, Saint-Martin C, Bouteiller D, LeGuern E, Apartis E, Rumbach L, Labauge P. Familial cortical myoclonic tremor with epilepsy (FCMTE): Clinical characteristics and exclusion of linkages to 8q and 2p in a large French family. *Rev Neurol* (Paris). 2009; 165: 812-820.

Labauge, P., Amer, L. O., Simonetta-Moreau, M., Attane, F., Tannier, C., Clanet, M., Castelnovo, G., An-Gourfinkel, I., Agid, Y., Brice, A., Ducros, A., LeGuern, E. Absence of linkage to 8q24 in a European family with familial adult myoclonic epilepsy (FAME). *Neurology* 58: 941-944, 2002. [PubMed: 11914412]

Madia F, Striano P, Di Bonaventura C, de Falco A, de Falco FA, Manfredi M, Casari G, Striano S, Minetti C, Zara F. Benign adult familial myoclonic epilepsy (BAFME): evidence of an extended founder haplotype on chromosome 2p11.1-q12.2 in five Italian families. *Neurogenetics* 2008; 9: 139-142.

Manabe Y, Narai H, Warita H, Hayashi T, Shiro Y, Sakai K, et al. Benign adult familial myoclonic epilepsy (BAFME) with night blindness. *Seizure* 2002; 11: 266–268.

Mikami M, Yasuda T, Terao A, Nakamura M, Ueno S, Tanabe H, Tanaka T, Onuma T, Goto Y, Kaneko S, Sano A. Localization of a gene for benign adult familial myoclonic epilepsy to chromosome 8q23.3-q24.1. *Am J Hum Genet* 1999; 65: 745-751.

Okino S. Familial benign myoclonus epilepsy of adult onset: a previously unrecognized myoclonic disorder. *J Neurol Sci* 1997; 145: 113-118.

Plaster NM, Uyama E, Uchino M, Ikeda T, Flanigan KM, Kondo I, Ptacek LJ. Genetic localization of the familial adult myoclonic epilepsy (FAME) gene to chromosome 8q24. *Neurology* 1999; 53: 1180-1183.

Regragui W, Gerdelat-Mas A, Simonetta-Moreau M. Cortical tremor (FCMTE: familial cortical myoclonic tremor with epilepsy). *Neurophysiol Clin* 2006; 36: 345-349.

Saka E, Saygi S. Familial adult onset myoclonic epilepsy associated with migraine. *Seizure* 2000; 9: 344–346.

Saint-Martin C, Bouteiller D, Stevanin G, Popescu C, Charon C, Ruberg M, Baulac S, LeGuern E, Labauge P, Depienne C. Refinement of the 2p11.1-q12.2 locus responsible for cortical tremor associated with epilepsy and exclusion of candidate genes. *Neurogenetics* 2008; 9: 69-71.

Schule B, Kock N, Svetel M, Dragasevic N, Hedrich K, de Carvalho Aguiar P, Liu L, Kabakci K, Garrels L, Meyer EM, Berisavac I, Schwinger E, Kramer PL, Ozelius LJ, Klein C, Kostic V. Genetic heterogeneity in ten families with myoclonus-dystonia. *J. Neurol Neurosurg Psychiat* 2004; 75: 1181-1185.

Striano P, de Falco FA, Minetti C, Zara F. Familial benign nonprogressive myoclonic epilepsies. *Epilepsia* 2009; 50(S5): 37-40.

Striano P, Madia F, Minetti C, Striano S, Zara F. Electroclinical and genetic findings in a family with cortical tremor, myoclonus and epilepsy. *Epilepsia.* 2005b; 46: 1993-5.

Striano P, Zara F, Striano S. Autosomal dominant cortical tremor, myoclonus and epilepsy:many syndromes, one phenotype. *Acta Neurologica Scandinavica* 2005a; 111: 211–217.

Suppa A, Berardelli A, Brancati F, Marianetti M, Barrano G, Mina C, Pizzuti A, Sideri G. Clinical, neuropsychological, neurophysiologic, and genetic features of a new Italian pedigree with familial cortical myoclonic tremor with epilepsy.*Epilepsia* 2009; 50: 1284-1288.

Terada K, Ikeda A, Mima T, Kimura M, Nagahama Y, Kamioka Y, Murone I, Kimura J, Shibasaki H. Familial cortical myoclonic tremor as a unique form of cortical reflex myoclonus. *Mov Disord* 1997; 12: 370–377.

Valente EM., Misbahuddin A, Brancati F, Placzek MR, Garavaglia B, Salvi S, Nemeth A, Shaw-Smith C, Nardocci N, Bentivoglio AR, Berardelli A, Eleopra R, Dallapiccola B, Warner TT. Analysis of the epsilon-sarcoglycan gene in familial and sporadic myoclonus-dystonia: evidence for genetic heterogeneity. *Mov Disord* 2003; 18: 1047-1051.

van Rootselaar AF, Aronica E, Steur ENHJ, Rozemuller-Kwakkel JM, de Vos RAI, Tijssen MAJ. Familial cortical tremor with epilepsy and cerebellar pathological findings. *Mov Disord* 2004; 19: 213-234.van Rootselaar, A.-F., Aronica, E., Steur, E. N. H. J., Rozemuller-Kwakkel, J. M., de Vos, R. A. I., Tijssen, M. A. J. Familial cortical tremor with epilepsy and cerebellar pathological findings. *Mov. Disord.* 19: 213-234, 2004. [PubMed: 14978679].

van Rootselaar, A.-F., van Schaik, I. N., van den Maagdenberg, A. M. J. M., Koelman, J. H. T. M., Callenbach, P. M. C., Tijssen, M. A. J. Familial cortical myoclonic tremor with epilepsy: a single syndromic classification for a group of pedigrees bearing common features. *Mov. Disord.* 20: 665-673, 2005. [PubMed: 15747356]

van Rootselaar F, Callenbach PMC, Hottenga JJ, Vermeulen FLMG, Speelman HD, Brouwer OF, Tijssen MAJ. A Dutch family with familial cortical tremor with epilepsy': clinical characteristics and exclusion of linkage to chromosome 8q23.3-q24.1. *J Neurol* 2002; 249: 829-834.

van Rootselaar AF, Maurits NM, Koelman JH, van der Hoeven JH, Bour LJ, Leenders KL, Brown P, Tijssen MA. Coherence analysis differentiates between cortical myoclonic tremor and essential tremor. *Mov Disord* 2006; 21: 215-22.

van Rootselaar AF, van Schaik IN, van den Maagdenberg AM JM, Koelman JHTM, Callenbach PMC, Tijssen MAJ. Familial cortical myoclonic tremor with epilepsy: a single syndromic classification for a group of pedigrees bearing common features. *Mov Disord* 2005; 20: 665-673.

van Rootselaar AF, van der Salm SM, Bour LJ, Edwards MJ, Brown P, Aronica E, Rozemuller-Kwakkel JM, Koehler PJ, Koelman JH, Rothwell JC, Tijssen MA. Decreased cortical inhibition and yet cerebellar pathology in familial cortical myoclonic tremor with epilepsy. *Mov Disord* 2007; 22: 2378-85.

Wakeno M. A family with heredofamilial tremor associated with epileptic disorders. *Seishin Shinkeigaku Zasshi* 1975; 77: 1–18.

In: Seizures and Anti-Epileptic Drugs
Editors: Willard Hosten and Aleph Burtsev
ISBN: 978-1-62100-255-0

Chapter VI

Pharmacogenomics of Antiepileptic Drug Therapy

Balraj Mittal[1*], Ritu Kumari[1], Ram Lakhan[1], R. K. Garg[3], J. Kalita[2] and U. K. Misra[2]

[1]Department of Genetics
[2]Neurology SGPGIMS, Lucknow, India
[3]Department of Neurology, CSMMU, Lucknow, India

Abstract

Epilepsy is the commonest serious neurological disorder worldwide. Despite multiple antiepileptic drug (AED) options, it has been established that 20-30% of epilepsies are not controlled by antiepileptic drugs. Drug resistance in epilepsy thus becomes an important clinical problem. The current developments in molecular medicine have led to the perspective that individual differences in responsiveness to drugs of various pharmacological classes, like many other human traits, are the result of a complex combination of genetic and environmental factors. According to this perspective, genes not only predispose to epilepsy but also determine responsiveness to antiepileptic drugs. Genetic variations of genes can potentially affect individual responsiveness to the drug at several steps that include drug absorption, drug distribution, drug metabolism, elimination and drug concentration at target sites. The metabolism of drug greatly influences its concentration in blood and target organ. The polymorphisms in the genes involved in drug metabolizing enzymes determine the drug levels in the plasma, thus affecting the effective dose and toxicity for antiepileptic drug. Some forms of idiopathic epilepsy have been found to be due to mutations in ion channels. There are also evidences of link between channel abnormalities and drug responsiveness in epilepsy. Several studies have documented association between drug transporter protein (MDR1 or ABCB1) genetic variants with drug resistance in epilepsy. Therefore, polymorphic genetic variants of drug metabolizing enzymes, multi drug transporters, receptors and ion channels are prime candidates for studies of drug responsiveness and

* E-mail addresses: balraj@sgpgi.ac.in, bml_pgi@yahoo.com (B. Mittal).

adverse drug reaction in epilepsy. In conclusion, new developments in pharmacogenomics hold great promise of antiepileptic drugs matched to specific genotypes.

Keywords: Pharmacogenetics, Polymorphisms, Interindividual Variations, Drug Metabolism, Drug Transport, Drug Targets, Personlized Medicine

Introduction

Epilepsy is a common but serious neurological disorder, which affects more than 60 million people worldwide (Szoeke *et al.,* 2006). Several pharmacological agents are available in the market for the treatment of epilepsy. In spite of best possible medications and treatment protocols, approximately one-third of patients do not respond adequately to anti epileptic drugs. Moreover, there is high incidence of adverse drug reactions (Engel *et al.*, 1998).Therefore, drug resistance and adverse drug reactions are important clinical problems in treatment of epilepsy. Large inter-individual variation in efficacy and adverse effects of anti-epileptic therapy presents opportunities and challenges in newly-emerging area of pharmacogenomics. The pharmacogenetics which is the study of interindividual variation in drug response and concept of ''personalized'' medicine are receiving much attention (de Leon, 2009). In recent years, expectations have been raised that pharmacogenetics may be an important tool to optimize the treatment of epilepsy for the individual patient or specific group of patients.

Pharmacogenetics and Drug Resistance in Epilepsy

Pharmacogenetics is the study of the impact of heritable traits on pharmacology and toxicology. Characterization of individual or population traits uses the principles of pharmacology and genetics to gain an understanding of the mechanism of human susceptibility to exogenous chemicals, including antiepileptic drugs (AEDs). An extension of pharmacogenetics is the discovery that genetic polymorphisms have the potential to affect a drug's mechanism of action. Actually, the interplay of genotype and drug efficacy has been defined as pharmacogenomics. In other words, we can say that genes not only predispose to epilepsy but are also believed to determine responsiveness to antiepileptic drugs. The study of individual genes whose variations exert a measurable influence on the effect of a given drug constitutes an important area of pharmacogenetics. Ever since genetic variability in drug metabolism was reported to affect the treatment with anti-epileptic drug phenytoin more than 25 years ago, the ultimate goal of pharmacogenetics is to use the genetic makeup of an individual to predict drug response and efficacy. The study of interindividual variation with respect to resistance to antiepileptic drugs (AEDs) i.e.; pharmacogenetic studies of epilepsy have received relatively little attention as compared other complex disorders and have not resulted in clinical application till date (Siddiqui *et al.*, 2003; Lakhan *et al.*, 2009; Szoeke *et al.*, 2009). The area of increasing genetic endeavor, "pharmacogenetics" is gaining concern, it is believed that it will finally lead to tailoring of medication including AEDs for each patient. In addition, pharmacogeneticists are also attempting to understand the genetic basis of refractory epilepsy so that they can identify subgroups of patients who share a common genetic background and then target drug therapies to meet their specific needs.

Candidate Genes in Pharmacogenetics of Epilepsy

In the post genomic era, the inter-individual variations in drug response have been attributed to allelic variations in genes (Wilson *et al.*, 2001; Jimenez *et al.*, 2003; Iafrate *et al.*, 2004). The genetic variations can potentially affect individual responsiveness to the drug at several steps, which include drug absorption, drug metabolism, drug transport, and drug targets (Figure 1).

There is growing list of polymorphisms found in different class of genes encoding drug metabolizing enzymes, drug transporters, receptors, and drug targets which have been linked to drug response in humans (Mc Corry *et al.*, 2004). Therefore, study of genetic variants of three classes of genes mentioned above are prime candidates for studies of drug responsiveness and adverse drug reaction in epilepsy.

Definition of Drug Resistance and Responsiveness

Failure to respond to AEDs is the usual basis for defining intractable epilepsy. Several investigators have proposed and used various definitions (Arts *et al.*, 1999; Berg *et al.*, 2003; Brodie, 2005; Berg and Kelly, 2006).

Additionally, it will remain important to continually reevaluate existing definitions of "drug resistance" as advances take place both in our understanding of the pathobiology of epilepsy and in the availability of newer AEDs. Patients who are considered drug resistant under a given definition may not remain so as newer antiepileptic drugs are developed, or designed, to target previously unappreciated underlying pathophysiological mechanisms. Though all definitions are significantly associated with longer-term outcome but no single preferred definition of intractable epilepsy exists. There needs to be consensus for a single definition of drug resistance in epilepsy so that results from different studies can be easily compared.

AED responders have typically been classified as anyone who is seizure free for >1 year to >2 years; non-responders as anyone who has one seizure/year to >10 seizures/year. Another criterion followed for multi-drug resistance is the occurrence of at least four seizures over a period of 1 year with three appropriate AEDs at maximum tolerated doses. The epilepsy patients who have complete freedom from seizures for at least 1 year from the last follow-up visit may be considered drug responsive. Given these widely different definitions, it is not surprising that some studies have found an association between specific genes and treatment resistance and others have not (Sisodiya and Marini., 2009).

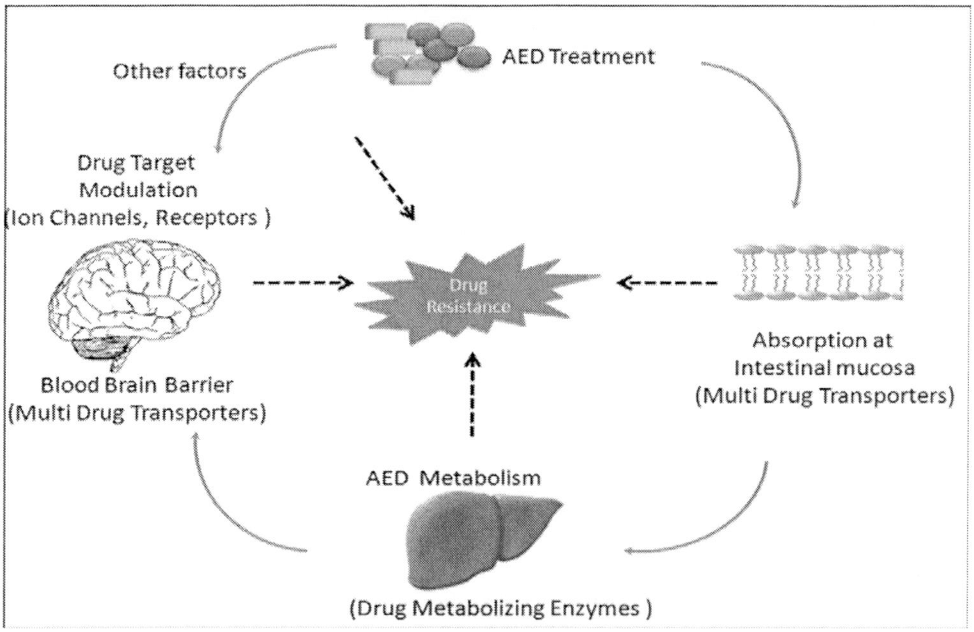

Figure 1. Schematic diagram showing factors which affects inter-individual variation and Drug resistance: Drug metabolizing enzymes (CYP2C9, 2C19, 3A4 and 2A6 etc); multi drug transporter (ABCB1, MRP1, MRP2 etc) and Drug Targets (ion channels and receptors e.g.; SCN2A, SCN1A, GABA and dopamine receptors).

Genetic Variations in Genes Related to Drug Metabolism

In pharmacotherapy; drug metabolism represents the primary pathway both in qualitative and quantitative elimination of drugs including AEDs. It is accomplished by the hepatic (metabolism) and/or renal (excretion) route which comprises phase I [(e.g., oxidative reactions catalyzed by various cytochrome P-450 enzymes (CYPs)] and phase II (e.g., conjugations like glucuronidation) reactions. CYP family comprises major phase-I drug metabolizing enzymes (DMEs), and is responsible for the metabolism of many commonly prescribed AEDs. Variants with very high enzymatic activity may be associated with a need for higher drug dosages than usually prescribed but low or absent biotransformation capacity may result in treatment failure due to inadequate drug levels (Ferraro and Buono., 2005). Similarly, variants with low enzymatic activities may result in build of higher levels of drug which can lead to potential toxicity of antiepileptic drugs (Eadie , 1991).

CYP family are major metabolisers of various commonly prescribe AEDs. In case of phenytoin (PHT) (a commonly prescribed AED), metabolism is stereoselective via p-hydroxylation to 4¢-OH-phenyl-5-phenylhydantoin (HPPH) by CYP2C9, but CYP2C19 is also involved in the formation of HPPH and secondary metabolites (Komatsu *et al.*, 2000). Various alleles of CYP2C9 and CYP2C19 exist in the populations and variant alleles have low or null enzyme activities. It was observed that the metabolic ratio (HPPH/PHT) was significantly lower in all mutant genotypes, if compared with the wild-type (CYP2C9*1/1).

Likewise, plasma levels of PHT were higher (up to 40%) in the subjects with mutant allele variants (van der Weide *et al.*, 2001). Carbamazepine (CBZ), another commonly used anti-epileptic drug, is primarily metabolized by CYP3A4 to its active CBZ-10, 11-epoxide, which subsequently is transformed by microsomal epoxide hydrolase (mEH) to the inactive CBZ-10, 11-diol, and finally is excreted into the urine in free and conjugated forms (Hata *et al.*, 2008; Kang *et al.*, 2008).

Metabolism of valproic acid (another AED) proceeds via three distinct pathways: (i) direct UDP mediated conjugation accounts for about 50% of a given dose, (ii) beta-oxidation accounts for about 40% and (iii) CYP mediated oxidation accounts for about 10% (Ketter *et al.*, 1999). Therefore, genetic variations can substantially contribute to inter-individual differences in AED therapies.

We carried out a study to evaluate the influence of CYP2C9 and CYP2C19 gene polymorphisms in multi-drug resistance phenotype in epilepsy patients from North India (Lakhan *et al.,* 2011). Our cohort included 402 epilepsy patients consisting of 274 patients who were drug responsive and 128 were drug resistant based on the criteria by Siddiqui *et al., 2003)*. The patient details including clinical characteristics are given in Table 1.

Genotyping was carried out from blood DNA, using PCR RFLP methodology. After analysis, none of the individuals (drug responsive or drug resistant epilepsy patients) were homozygous for the *2C9*2* (430 C >T) or *2C9*3*(1075 A>C). No significant differences were observed at allele level for *2C9*2* 430 T variant (OR = 0.67, 95% CI = 0.28-0.1.50, P=0.36). *CYP2C9* 1075 A>C (*3 variant) polymorphism showed marginal significant difference between patients having multiple drug resistance and drug responsive patients for AC genotype (OR = 0.57, 95%CI=0.32-1.00; P=0.05).

The *CYP2C9**3 variant allele frequency was also bit higher in drug responsive patients compared to drug resistant patients (P=0.06; OR = 0.60, 95%CI=0.35-1.03) and appeared to be contributing towards lower risk for developing multiple drug resistance in epilepsy (Figure 2). For CYP2C19, *2 did not show any significant association with AED treatment and CYP2C19*3 was monomorphic in our population.

In our present study, we observed the protective effects of mutant alleles of *CYP2C9*2* (430 C>T) and *CYP2C9*3* (1075 A>C) in epilepsy patients developing multiple drug resistance. These findings indicate important role of *CYP2C9* variants in conferring multiple-drug resistant phenotype against AEDs.

The results are also in support of previous observations which identified *CYP2C9* as major drug metabolizer for commonly prescribed AEDs (Aynacioglu *et al.*, 1999). *CYP2C9* is responsible for the hydroxylation of up to 90% of serum phenytoin. Among AEDs, phenytoin, carbamazepine and phenobarbital mainly undergo significant metabolism by cytochrome P450 isozymes.

Earlier studies have also observed strong association between *CYP2C9* genotype and phenytoin maintenance dose requirement (Weide *et al., 2001).* found that *CYP2C9* allelic variants affect phenytoin dose requirement; for patients carrying at least one mutant *CYP2C9* allele, the mean phenytoin dose required to achieve a therapeutic serum concentration was about 37% lower than the mean dose required by wild-type individuals.

Another similar study from Taiwan revealed that the *CYP2C9* and *CYP2C19* polymorphisms have dramatic effects on the population pharmacokinetic parameters of phenytoin.

Table 1. Characteristic profile of drug responsive and drug resistant epilepsy patients

Sex		Drug Responsive (258)	Drug Resistant (127)
Male		186(72.1%)	97(76.4%)
Female		72(27.9%)	30(23.6%)
Age (years)±SD		24.52 ± 11.31	23.61 ± 11.73
Age of Onset		17.09 ± 10.51	14.68 ± 10.24
AED therapy at the last clinic visit			
Monotherapy		169 (28.8%)	
Polytherapy		216 (36.8%)	
Classification			
Localization related epilepsy and syndrome	Idiopathic localization related epilepsy	23(8.9%)	14(11%)
	Symptomatic localization related epilepsy	130(50.4%)	74(58.3%)
Generalized epilepsy and syndrome	Idiopathic generalized epilepsy	102(39.5%)	35(27.6%)
	Symptomatic generalized epilepsy	3(1.2%)	4(3.1%)

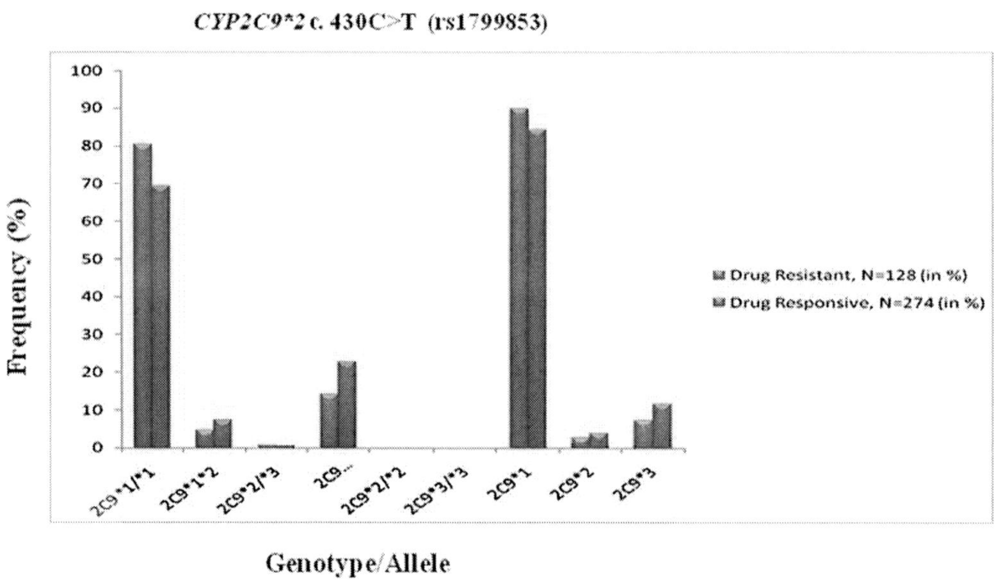

Figure 2. Distribution of CYP2C9 genetic variants: Genotype and allele frequencies in epilepsy patient between drug resistant and drug responsive group.

On the basis of these observations, we propose that poor metabolizer phenotype could have advantage over extensive metabolizer phenotype in epilepsy pharmacotherapy; it is likely that patients with poor metabolizer phenotype will require lesser drug doses to control seizures as compared to epilepsy patients with extensive metabolism. So, patients with extensive metabolism are more likely to become drug resistant during the course of antiepileptic treatment (Lakhan *et al.*, 2011, Kumari et al, 2011a).

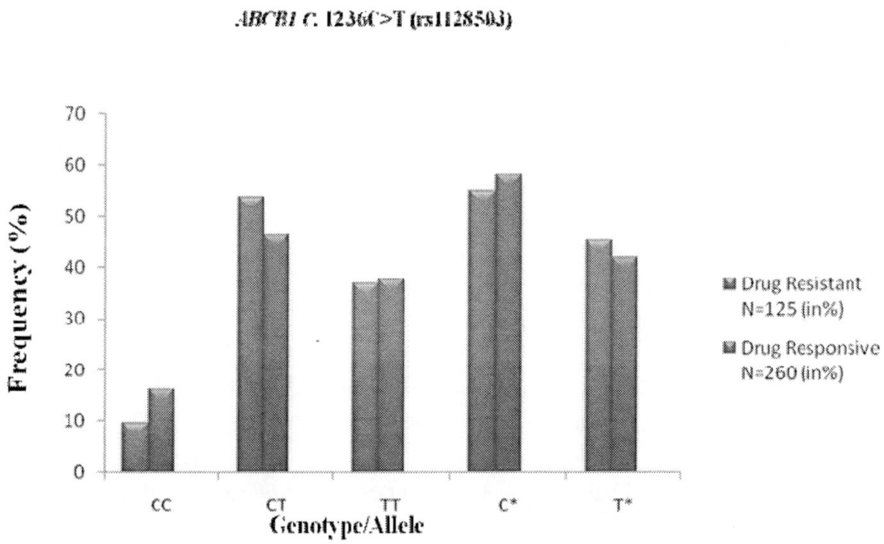

Figure 3. Distribution of *ABCB1;* 1236C>T (rs1128503) gene polymorphisms in drug resistant and drug responsive epilepsy patients.

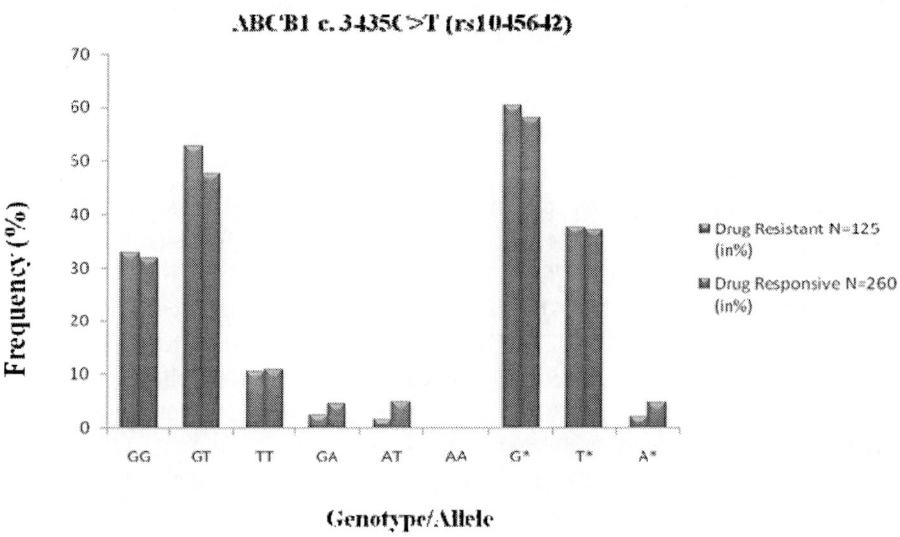

Figure 4. Distribution of ABCB1; 3435C>T (rs1045642) gene polymorphism in drug resistant and responsive patients with epilepsy.

Genetic Variations in Genes Related to Drug Transport

Several classes of drug transport proteins are also known to have pharmacogenetic relevance. The solute carrier (SLC) proteins and ATP-binding cassette family proteins are prime candidates for such studies. These diverse classes of transporters include organic anion transporters, organic cation transporters, dipeptide transporters, nucleoside transporters etc. (Gerloff, 2004). The *ABCB1* (MDR1) gene codes for prototype molecule p-glycoprotein (p-GP) that is considered a key element in regulating access of a diverse array of therapeutic agents to the brain and other tissues.

Most antiepileptic drugs are planar lipophilic agents and thus many of them are substrates for the ABCB1 membrane transporter and P-glycoprotein), the up regulation of which is a well known cause of multidrug-resistance phenotype in anti-cancer therapy (Ling ,1997). These membrane transporter proteins actively extrude drugs from cells, with the potential to affect both toxicity and efficacy. In drug refractory patients with epilepsy, the multidrug-resistance phenotype has been associated with increased ABCB1 levels in resected brain tissue (Tishler *et al.*, 1995; Lazarowski *et al.*, 1999; Dombrowski *et al.*, 2001; Sisodiya *et al.*, 2002; Ak *et al.*, 2007). The ATP-binding cassette subfamily B member 1 (ABCB1) proteins are products of multidrug resistance (MDR) genes that are expressed widely and also constitute the blood–brain barrier responsible for ATP-mediated efflux of different compounds outside the brain and serve as a defense mechanism. Over expression of P-gp has been reported in endothelial cells isolated from temporal lobe blood vessels of medically intractable epilepsy patients. A number of studies from different populations have explored the role of these polymorphisms in *ABCB1* genes on drug refractory epilepsy but have shown conflicting results. A large number of studies have evaluated the role of ABCB1 gene polymorphisms in drug resistance phenotype in different populations but results are still conflicting. We also performed a case control association study to evaluate the influence of three most commonly studied polymorphisms- *ABCB1*3435C>T, 1236C>T and 2677G>T/A in a cohort of epilepsy patients from North India. We used inclusion criteria for responder and non-responders which were similar and consistent with original study by Siddiqui *et al.*, 2003). The results of the study are depicted in Figure 3 to Figure 5 (Lakhan et al, 2009a).

The genotype frequencies of *ABCB1* 3435C>T did not differ significantly in drug resistant versus responsive patients for CT (P=0.06; OR=1.95; 95% CI=0.96-3.96) and TT (P=0.18; OR=1.64; 95% CI=0.79-3.41) genotypes (Figure 3). No significant differences were observed at allele level also (P= 0.39; OR = 1.14; 95% CI = 0.84-1.54). In *ABCB1 c.2* 677G>A polymorphism, allele 'A' was associated with drug resistant phenotype in epilepsy patients (P = 0.03, OR = 0.31, 95% CI = 0.10–0.93). However, genotype frequencies of 2677G>T *ABCB1* polymorphism did not differ significantly in drug resistant versus drug responsive epilepsy patients for GT genotype (P=0.71; OR = 1.14, 95% CI=0.55-2.36), for TT genotype (P= 0.87; OR = 1.06; 95% CI 0.49-2.26) and for AT genotype (P= 0.39; OR = 0.53; 95%; CI= 0.13-2.24) (Figure 4). Similarly, genotype and allele frequencies of 1236C>T *ABCB1* polymorphism also did not differ significantly in drug resistant and responsive groups for CT (P=0.32; OR = 1.40; 95% CI=0.62-2.61), and TT (P= 0.50; OR = 1.27; 95% CI=0.77-1.42) genotypes (Figure 5). Haplotypes were constructed for the three SNPs of ABCB1 gene but none of the haplotypes showed significant difference between drug resistant and drug responsive patients (Figure 6).

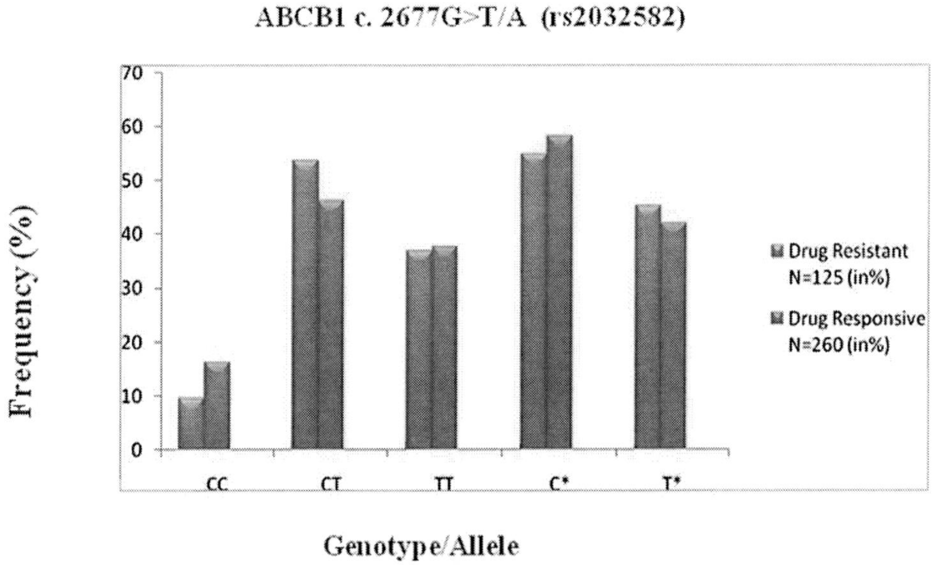

Figure 5. Distribution of ABCB1; 2677G>T/A (rs2032582) gene polymorphism in drug resistant and responsive patients with epilepsy.

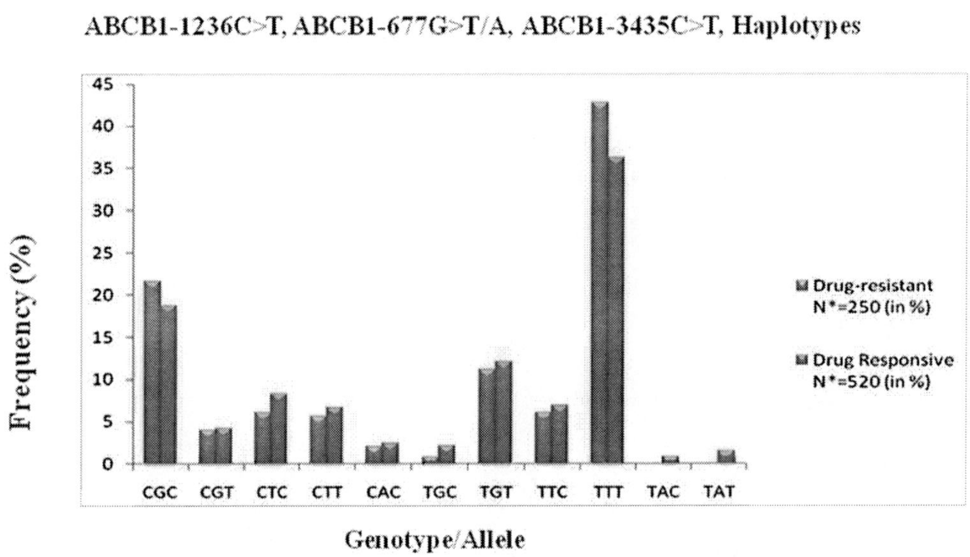

Figure 6. Distribution of Haplotype frequencies of ABCB1-1236C>T, ABCB1-677G>T/A, ABCB1-3435C>T, gene polymorphisms in drug resistant and drug responsive epilepsy patient.

Many factors may be attributed for non-uniformity and non-replication of results from various studies. These include low sample size and genetic heterogeneity within groups. Also, as mentioned earlier, there is no consensus on single definition of intractability. Individual studies use different definitions, creating difficulties for comparisons of results across studies. Moreover, it is now accepted that drug resistance is a complex phenotype, resulting from contribution of numerous other genes in addition to drug metabolizing enzymes, and drug transporters (Sisodiya and Marini, 2009). Moreover, clinical studies of this gene and its different variants have thus far been done only on retrospective cohorts and in patients with chronic epilepsy undergoing treatment at tertiary care centers. Though study of drug transporter genes has potential to affect responsiveness in AED therapy via efflux mechanisms but needs further investigations.

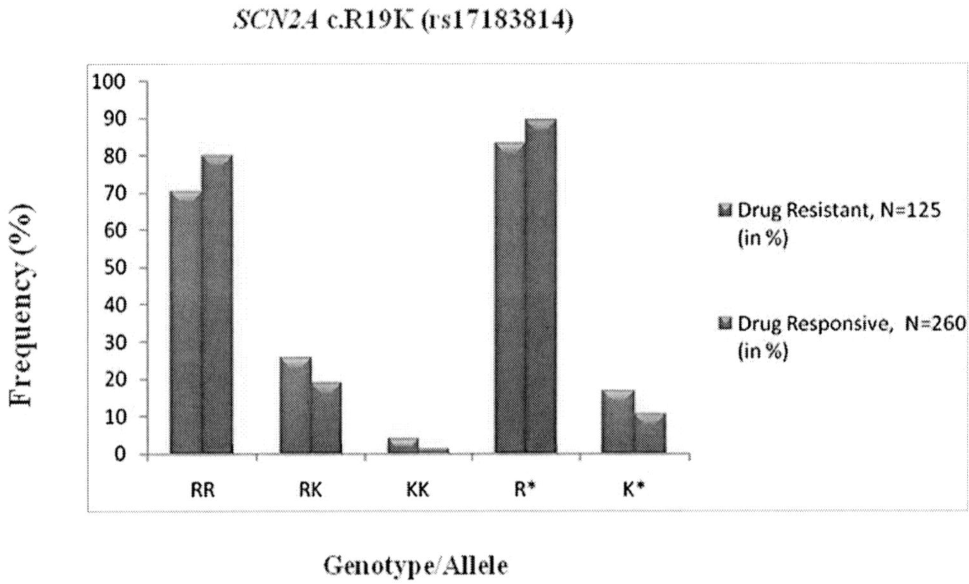

Figure 7. Distribution of SCN2A genetic polymorphism (rs17183814) Genotype and allele frequencies in epilepsy patient between drug resistant and drug responsive group.

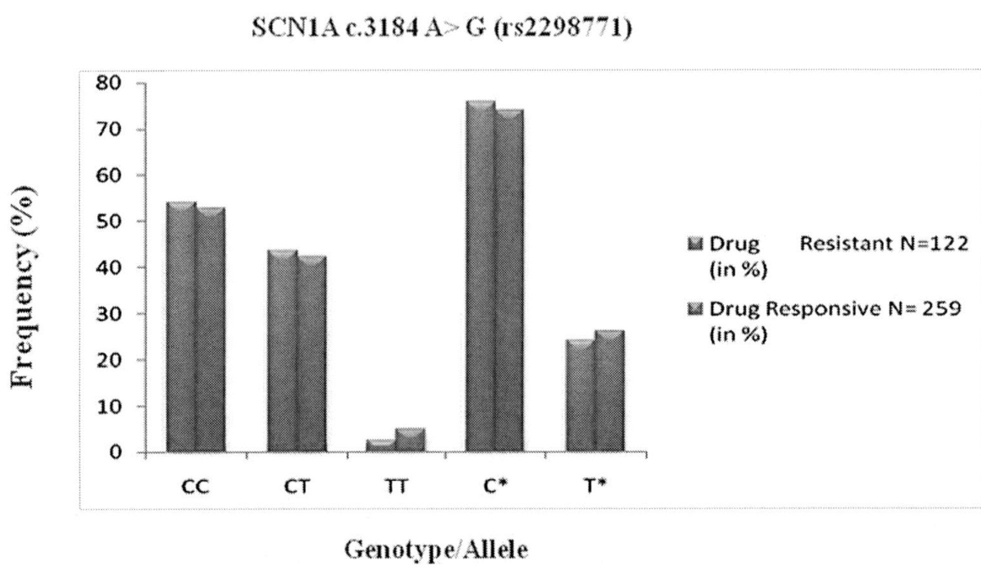

Figure 8. Distribution of SCN1A; c.3184 A> G (rs2298771) gene polymorphism in drug resistant and responsive patients with epilepsy.

Genetic Variations in Genes Related to Drug Targets

The role of voltage-gated and ligand-gated ion channels in epileptogenesis, and as targets in the development of new antiepileptic drugs (AEDs) is very important (Armijo *et al.*, 2005). The most common targets of AEDs identified are voltage-gated sodium channels high voltage-gated calcium channels and ligand-gated neurotransmitter receptors (Mulley *et al*, 2003). Voltage-gated Na+ channels are essential for action potentials, and their mutations have been identified in generalized epilepsy with febrile seizures plus and benign familial neonatal infantile seizures. In addition, many new genes like synapsin may be associated with idiopathic epilepsy and may also be explored for their role the drug response (Lakhan et al, 2009).

Voltage-Gated Sodium Channels

Voltage dependent sodium channels are heterologous multisubunit complexes that contain a large 'a' subunit and two smaller 'b' subunits. The sodium channels are generally recognized as the major target with respect to antiepileptic efficacy (Rogawski and Loscher., 2004). Phenytoin has been well documented to block voltage- dependent sodium channels, and this is generally regarded as its primary mechanism of action. As for most drugs that interact with ion channels, the action of phenytoin is complex. Nonetheless, there is some agreement that the primary action of phenytoin involves binding to a subunit of the sodium channel in its inactivated state (Catterall, 2000). This property contributes to the ability of phenytoin and related drugs to selectively inhibit repetitive high-frequency spike ring of neurons. Based on this known molecular action of phenytoin, previous study by Tate et al (2005) reported significant association between an intronic polymorphism in the SCN1A gene and maximum doses of both carbamazepine and phenytoin. It was shown that the polymorphism disrupts the consensus sequence of the 5'-splice donor site of a highly conserved alternative exon, and it significantly affects the proportions of the alternative transcripts in individuals with a history of epilepsy (Tate *et al.*, 2005). This study is especially noteworthy, as it is the first reported genetic association between an antiepileptic drug and a pharmacodynamic target protein. Sodium channel a subunit, SCN2A, is also a target for phenytoin binding (Xie *et al*, 2001) and polymorphism of the gene encoding this protein also warrants study in relation to the effects of phenytoin treatment in epilepsy patients. Specific amino acid residues at positions 1764 (Phe) and 1771 (Tyr) have been identified as constituting part of a common binding site for phenytoin and other drugs that interact with voltage-dependent sodium channels (Ragsdale *et al.*, 1996), and these data provide the basis for focused, testable hypotheses with respect to mechanisms underlying individual differences in responsiveness to phenytoin. Like phenytoin, carbamazepine and its derivative oxcarbazepine block voltage-gated sodium channels. Carbamazepine binds to a common site on the 'a' subunit of sodium channels shared with phenytoin and lamotrigine (Kuo, 1998). Due to differences in chemical structure, carbamazepine and phenytoin exhibit quantitative differences with respect to channel binding affinity and the kinetics of binding (Kuo,1998).

Nonetheless, given their shared molecular mechanism, carbamazepine and phenytoin are subject to similar pharmacogenetic influences. Thus, as described above, variation in the SCNA1 sodium channel subunit gene is associated with individual differences in responsiveness to both carbamazepine and phenytoin (Tate *et al*, 2005). Such overlapping mechanisms of action suggest that there may be shared genetic influences across larger groups of antiepileptic drugs, and the design of future pharmacogenetic studies may allow for such hypotheses to be tested.

Sodium Ion channel Gene Polymorphisms in Drug Resistance Epilepsy

Until now, very few studies have correlated drug targets like sodium channels in drug resistance and therapeutic dosage in patients with epilepsy. Therefore, we looked for an association of the polymorphisms in SCN1A and SCN2A genes with drug resistance phenotype in our patient groups from North India. Even though *SCN1A* c.3184 A>G polymorphism was associated with generalized epilepsy, it showed no influence on multidrug resistance phenotype in patients with epilepsy. Similarly, (Kwan *et al..2008).* also found no involvement of this polymorphism in drug resistance epilepsy. However, *SCN1A* IVS5–91 G>A intronic polymorphism of same gene has been reported to show population-specific association with carbamazepine and multiple drug resistance epilepsy (Tate *et.al.*,2005,2006, Abe *et.al.*,2008).

The genotype or allelic frequencies of *SCN1A* c.A3184G polymorphism in our study group did not differ significantly in drug-resistant *vs.* drug-responsive epilepsy patients for AG (P = 0.98; OR 0.99, 95% CI 0.62- 1.58) or GG (P = 0.78; OR 1.17 95% CI 036- 3.78) (Figure 7). Similarly, genotype frequencies of *SCN2A* c.R19K also did not differ significantly in drug resistant versus responsive patients for RK (P=0.97; OR=1.44; 95% CI=0.84–2.48) and KK (P=0.09; OR=3.49; 95%CI=0.81-14.97) genotypes (Figure 8). However, frequency of K allele was significantly higher in drug resistant patients with epilepsy versus drug responsive patients (P=0.03; OR 1.62 95% CI=1.03-2.56). It suggests *SCN2A* c.R19K polymorphism may be involved in modulating drug response in epilepsy patients (Lakhan et al, 2009b, Kumari et al, 2011a).

$GABA_A$ Receptor Gene Polymorphisms in Drug Resistance Epilepsy

GABA (γ-amino butyric acid) receptors have always been an inviting target in the etiology and treatment of epilepsy because of its role as a major inhibitory neurotransmitter in the brain. It acts through three receptor classes; the ionotropic $GABA_A$, $GABA_C$ receptors and the metabotropic $GABA_B$ receptors. Among the three receptors, recent findings highlight the significance of $GABA_A$ receptor heterogeneity for the concept of E/I (excitation /inhibition) balance and its relevance for epilepsy (Fritschy et al., 2008).

In the 1970s, understanding the role of GABA as an inhibitory neurotransmitter in the brain led to the design of compounds that would modify the disposition of GABA so as to increase its inhibitory activity and thereby protect against seizures. Thus, seizures occur in animals and humans if GABA synthesis is impaired (as in pyridoxine deficiency or by exposure to isoniazid, a pyridoxine antagonist) or if GABAA receptors are inhibited by any one of a diverse group of compounds such as bicuculline, PTZ, picrotoxin, penicillin, convulsant barbiturates, and inverse benzodiazepine-site ligands. AEDs such as benzodiazepines, phenobarbital, gabapentin and topiramate are important targets of $GABA_A$ receptor (Mosche , 2000).

GABA operates primarily via chloride-permeable $GABA_A$ receptor channels. From a genetic perspective, all mutations documented to date are localized to $GABA_A$ receptors rather than $GABA_B$ and $GABA_C$ receptors. Structurally, $GABA_A$ receptors are pentameric chloride ion channels formed from various combinations of proteins encoded by α (α 1– α 6), β (β 1– β 3), γ (γ 1– γ 3); δ, ε, θ, and ρ (ρ1– ρ3) subunit gene families (Reid *et al*., 2009). Numerous experimental and clinical observations suggest that epilepsy may result from an imbalance in excitatory and inhibitory neurotransmitter systems resulting in decreased net inhibition.

Conventional antiepileptic drugs (e.g. barbiturates, benzodiazepines) suppress seizures by increasing $GABA_A$ receptor activity, or by inhibition of GABA breakdown (vigabatrin) or reuptake (tiagabin) (Loscher *et al.,2004)*. It is also hypothesized that, target receptor sites are somehow altered in epileptic brain so that they are much less sensitive to anticonvulsive effects of administered antiepileptic drugs (Mosche *et al*., 2000). These receptors are also key therapeutic targets for benzodiazepines, barbiturates, neurosteroids and general anesthetics (Moult et al., 2010).

Genetic variations in genes encoding GABA receptors have been shown to bring about inter-individual variation in susceptibility to various neurological syndromes including schizopherenia, epilepsy and alcohol-withdrawal syndromes.

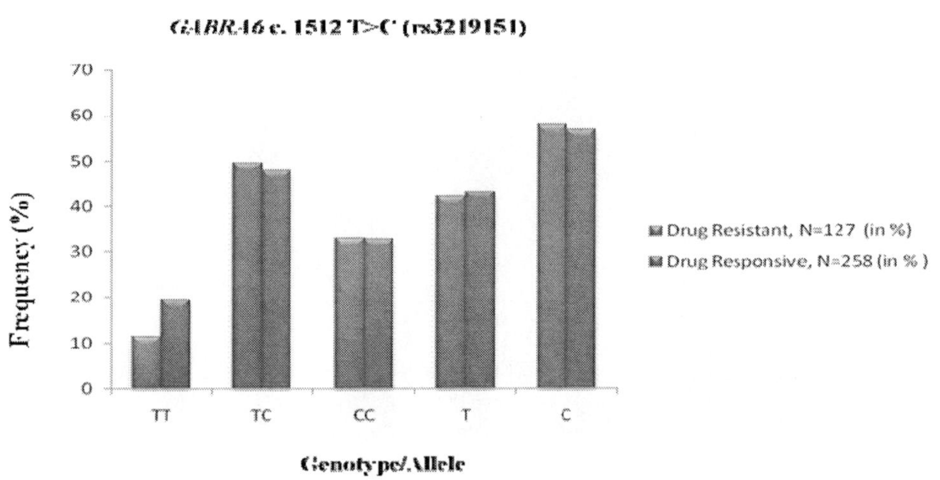

Figure 9. Distribution of GABRA6 (rs3219151) polymorphism in drug resistant and responsive patients with epilepsy.

Our present study was designed to evaluate the association of $GABA_A$ receptor subunit subtypes variants *GABRA1* IVS11 + 15 A > G, *GABRG2* 588C > T, *GABRA6* c. 1512 T>C (rs3219151), *GABRB2 c.* 1412 C>T (rs2229944), and *GABRR2 c.* IVS2 C>G (rs9362632) gene polymorphisms with epilepsy susceptibility and pharmacotherapy in north Indian epilepsy patients (Kumari *et al.*, 2010, 2011b). We observed significant differences at genotype as well as allele frequencies of *GABRA1 A > G* polymorphism in drug resistant versus drug responsive epilepsy patients for homozygous variant GG genotype (P = 0.03, OR = 1.84, 95% CI = 1.05–3.23) and G allele (P = 0.02, OR = 1.43, 95% CI = 1.05–1.95) (Figure 9).

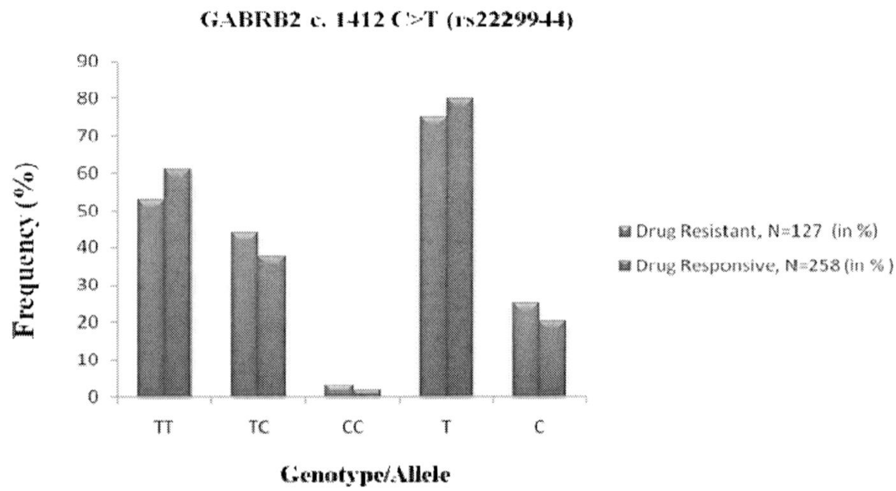

Figure 10. Distribution of GABRB2 (rs2229944) polymorphism in drug resistant and responsive patients with epilepsy.

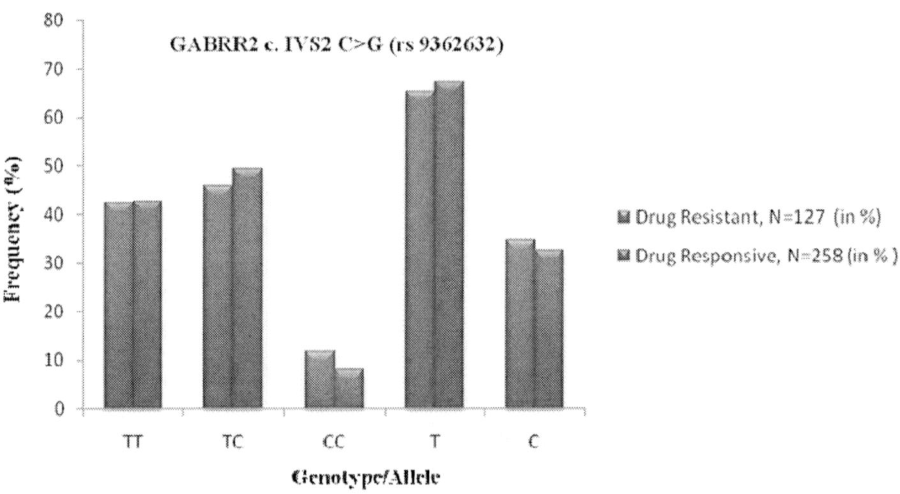

Figure 11. Distribution of GABRR2 (rs9362632) polymorphism in drug resistant and responsive patients with epilepsy.

However, none of the genetic variants of *GABRG2* 588C > T, *GABRA6* c. 1512 T>C (rs3219151), *GABRB2 c.* 1412 C>T (rs2229944), and *GABRR2 c.* IVS2 C>G (rs9362632) show any significant differences in drug resistant versus drug responsive epilepsy patients either at genotype or allele levels (Figure 10 to Figure 13). It suggests that except *GABRA1* IVS11 + 15 A > G intronic polymorphism, other variants may not be involved in drug response in epilepsy patients.

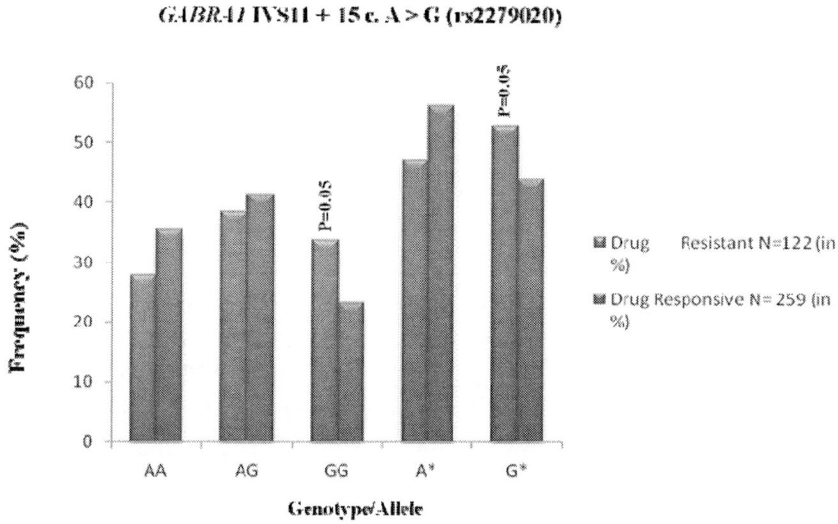

Figure 12. Distribution of GABRA1; IVS11 + 15 A > G (rs2279020) gene polymorphism in drug-resistant and -responsive patients with epilepsy (Kumari et.al.,2011).

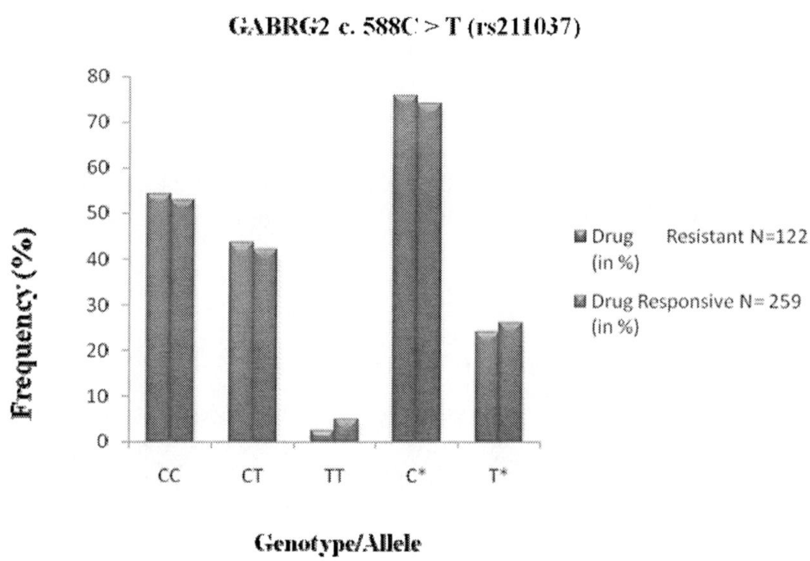

Figure 13. Distribution of *GABRG2* c.588C > T (rs211037) gene polymorphism in drug-resistant and -responsive patients with epilepsy (Kumari et.al., 2010).

It is possible that the association of *GABRA1* IVS11 + 15 A > G polymorphism with refractory phenotype in our study may be due to changes in the structure and function of inhibitory $GABA_A$ receptors (Kumari *et al.,* 2010). Excessive glutamate excitation and activation of drug resistance genes may also contribute to changes in GABA receptor conformation and loss of drug efficacy.

Discussion

In the post genomic era, the inter-individual variations in drug response have been attributed to allelic variations in genes. Multiple genes are known to be responsible for drug responsiveness, for example drug metabolizing enzymes (Nelson *et al.,* 2004) include mainly cytochrome P450, drug transporters (MDR1) and drug targets which include sodium channels, potassium channels, and GABA receptors.

In the above mentioned facts, we have provided evidence that genetic variations in all three classes of genes have some role in multiple drug resistance; but it would be desirable to replicate them in larger cohorts. It should also be kept in mind that over all genetic effect of these genes may have greater role in determining drug responsiveness rather than a single gene and its genetic polymorphisms alone. Response to newly administered AED treatments is highly dependent on past treatment history. Other factors such as type of epilepsy, duration of seizure, and number of seizures prior to initiation of drug therapy. may also be responsible for differences in drug responsiveness.

It may be kept in mind that epilepsy is a heterogenous condition with multiple etiologies, the pathogenesis of AED resistance is multifactorial and may involve both genetic and environmental factors (Kim *et.al.,* 2011).The current studies associating particular genes and their variants with seizure control or adverse events have inherent weaknesses, yet it is believed that pharmacogenomic studies with clearly defined phenotypes involving multicenter approach will result in therapeutic application.

In future, newer genetic methodologies, in particular genomewide association studies (GWAS) capable of examining millions of human single nucleotide polymorphism in thousands of individuals, combined with robust novel phenotypes in large multicentre collaborations should permit substantial progress in understanding the genetic basis of drug resistance and perhaps identify new targets for therapy of drug-resistant epilepsy (Sisodiya and Marini, 2009).

Clinical Translation

The use of genotyping to informed clinical decisions about drug use is not widely practiced. The slow pace of the clinical application of pharmacogenomics has many reasons. Obviously, the most important issue is the need to establish clinical utility in order to support the value of genotyping. So far, there seems to be little consensus among researchers on the level or nature of data required to establish clinical utility (Woodcock ,2010).

In addition, physicians and other health care providers need to be aware of this area of biomedical science in order to apply the information clinically. A major effort will be required to educate all members of the health care team about clinical genomics (Wang ,et al.,, 2011) In long term perspective, the pharmacogenomic knowledge will help our pharmaceutical industry to develop drugs, which are more suited to the people of the country. The clinical trial data for newer antiepileptic drugs will be more relevant if data on the genomic profile of different populations is available.

References

Abe T, Seo T, Ishitsu T, Nakagawa T, Hori M, Nakagawa K. Association between SCN1A polymorphism and carbamazepine-resistant epilepsy. *Br J Clin Pharmacol.* 2008;(66):304–7.

Ak H, Ay B, Tanriverdi T, Sanus GZ, Is M, Sar M, Oz B, Ozkara C, Ozyurt E and Uzan M. Expression and cellular distribution of multidrug resistance-related proteins in patients with focal cortical dysplasia. *Seizure.*2007;(16):493-503.

Armijo JA, Shushtarian M, Valdizan EM, Cuadrado A, de las Cuevas I et al , Ion channels and epilepsy. *Curr Pharm Des.* 2005;11(15):1975-2003.

Arts WF, Geerts AT, Brouwer OF, Boudewyn Peters AC, Stroink H and van Donselaar CA. The early prognosis of epilepsy in childhood: the prediction of a poor outcome. The Dutch study of epilepsy in childhood. *Epilepsia.*1999;(40):726-734.

Aynacioglu AS, Brockmoller J, Bauer S, Sachse C, Guzelbey P, Ongen Z, Nacak M. and Roots I. Frequency of cytochrome P450 CYP2C9 variants in a Turkish population and functional relevance for phenytoin. *Br J Clin Pharmacol.*1999;(48):409-415.

Berg AT and Kelly MM. Defining Intractability: Comparisons among Published Definitions. *Epilepsia.*2006;(47):431-436.

Berg AT, Vickrey BG, Langfitt JT, Sperling MR, Walczak TS, Shinnar S, Bazil CW, Pacia SV and Spencer SS. The multicenter study of epilepsy surgery: recruitment and selection for surgery. *Epilepsia.*2003;(44):1425-1433.

Brodie MJ.Diagnosing and predicting refractory epilepsy. *Acta Neurol Scand Suppl.* 2005;(181):36-39.

Catterall WA. From ionic currents to molecular mechanisms: the structure and function of voltage-gated sodium channels. *Neuron.* 2000;(26): 13-25.

de Leon J, Pharmacogenomics: The promise of personalized medicine for CNS disorders. *Neuropsychopharmacology.*2009;(34):159-172.

Dombrowski SM, Desai SY, Marroni M, Cucullo L, Goodrich K, Bingaman W, Mayberg MR, Bengez L and Janigro D. Overexpression of Multiple Drug Resistance Genes in Endothelial Cells from Patients with Refractory Epilepsy. *Epilepsia* 2001;(42):1501-1506.

Eadie MJ. Formation of active metabolites of anticonvulsant drugs: a review of their pharmacokinetic and therapeutic significance. *Clin Pharmacokinet.*1991;(21):27-41.

Engel, J.Classifications of the International League Against Epilepsy: time for reappraisal. *Epilepsia.*1998;(39): 1014-1017.

Ferraro TN, Buono RJ. The relationship between the pharmacology of antiepileptic drugs and human gene variation: An overview. *Epilepsy Behavior.* 2005;(7): 18-36.

Fritschy J M. Epilepsy, E/I Balance and GABA(A) Receptor plasticity. *Front Mol Neurosci.*2008; (1):5.

Gerloff T. Impact of genetic polymorphisms in transmembrane carrier-systems on drug and xenobiotic distribution. *Naunyn Schmiedebergs Arch Pharmacol.*2004;(369):69-77.

Hata M, Tanaka Y, Kyoda N, Osakabe T, Yuki H, Ishii I, Kitada M, Neya S and Hoshino T. An epoxidation mechanism of carbamazepine by CYP3A4. *Bioorg Med Chem.* 2008;(16): 5134-5148.

Iafrate AJ, Feuk L, Rivera MN, Listewnik ML, Donahoe PK, Qi Y, Scherer SW, Lee C. Detection of large-scale variation in the human genome. *Nature Genetics.* 2004;(36): 949-51.

Jimenez-Sanchez G. Developing a platform for genomic medicine in Mexico. *Science.* 2003; (300): 295-6.

Kang P, Liao M, Wester MR, Leeder JS, Pearce RE and Correia MA. CYP3A4-Mediated carbamazepine (CBZ) metabolism: formation of a covalent CBZ-CYP3A4 adduct and alteration of the enzyme kinetic profile. *Drug Metab Dispos.*2008;(36):490-499.

Ketter TA, Frye MA, Cora-Locatelli G, Kimbrell TA and Post RM. Metabolism and excretion of mood stabilizers and new anticonvulsants. *Cell Mol Neurobiol.*1999;(19):511-532.

Kim MK, Jason H Moore JH, Kim JK, Cho KH, Cho YW, Kim YS,Lee MC, Kim YO and Shin MH Evidence for epistatic interactions in antiepileptic drug resceistan. *J Human Genet.*2011; (56): 71–76.

Komatsu T, Yamazaki H, Asahi S, Gillam EM, Guengerich FP, Nakajima M and Yokoi T.Formation of a dihydroxy metabolite of phenytoin in human liver microsomes/cytosol: roles of cytochromes P450 2C9, 2C19, and 3A4. *Drug Metab Dispos.* 2000;(28):1361-1368.

Kumari R, Lakhan R, Kalita J, Misra UK, Mittal B. Association of alpha subunit of GABAA receptor subtype gene polymorphisms with epilepsy susceptibility and drug resistance in north Indian population. *Seizure.*2010;(19):237-41.

Kumari R, Lakhan R, Garg RK, Kalita J, Misra UK, Mittal B. Pharmacogenomic association study on the role of drug metabolizing, drug transporters and drug target gene polymorphisms in drug-resistant epilepsy in a north Indian population. *Ind J Hum Gen,*2011a (17) Suppl 1:S32-40.

Kumari R, Lakhan R, Kalita J, Garg RK, Misra UK, Mittal B. Potential role of GABAA receptor subunit; GABRA6, GABRB2 and GABRR2 gene polymorphisms in epilepsy susceptibility and pharmacotherapy in North Indian population. *Clinica Chimica Acta,* 2011b;(412):1244-1248.

Kuo CC. A common anticonvulsant binding site for phenytoin, carbamazepine, and lamotrigine in neuronal Na+ channels. *Mol Pharmacol.* 1998;(54):712–21.

Kwan P, Poon WS, Ng HK, Kang DE,Wong V, Ng PW, Lui CH, Sin NC,Wong KS, Baum L. Multidrug resistance in epilepsyand polymorphisms in the voltage-gated sodium channelgenes SCN1A, SCN2A, and SCN3A: correlation amongphenotype, genotype, and mRNA expression. *Pharmacogenet Genomics.* 2008;(18):989-98.

Lakhan R, Kumari R, Misra UK, Kalita J, Pradhan S. and Mittal B. Differential Role of Sodium channels SCN1A and SCN2A gene polymorphisms with epilepsy and multiple drug resistance in north Indian population. *Brit J Clin Pharmacol.* 2009;(68):214-220.

Lakhan R, Misra UK, Kalita J, et al. No association of ABCB1 polymorphisms with drug-refractory epilepsy in a north Indian population. *Epilepsy Behav.* 2009;(14):78–82.

Lakhan R, Kalita J, Misra UK, Kumari R and Mittal B. Association of intronic polymorphism rs3773364 A>G in synapsin-2 gene with idiopathic epilepsy. *Synapse,*2009;(64): 403-408.

Lakhan R, Kumari R, Singh K, Misra UK, Kalita J, Mittal B, Possible role of *CYP2C9* and *CYP2C19* single nucleotide polymorphisms in drug refractory Epilepsy.*Ind J Med Res,* 2011; (In press).

Lazarowski A, Sevlever G, Taratuto A, Massaro M and Rabinowicz A. Tuberous sclerosis associated with MDR1 gene expression and drug-resistant epilepsy. *Pediatr Neurol.*1999;(21):731-734.

Ling V. Multidrug resistance: molecular mechanisms and clinical relevance. *Cancer Chemother Pharmacol.1997*;(40):Suppl, S3-8.

Loscher W, Schmidt D. New horizons in the development of antiepileptic drugs:the search for new targets. *Epilepsy Res.* 2004;(60):77–159.

McCorry D, Chadwick D, and Marson A. Current drug treatment of epilepsy in adults. *Lancet Neurol.* 2004 ;(3): 729-35.

Meldrum BS and MA. Molecular targets for antiepileptic drug development. *Neurotherapeutics* 2007; 4:18–61.

Moshe SL. Mechanisms of action of anticonvulsant agents. *Neurology.* 2000;(55): S32–40 [discussion S54-38].

Moult PR. Neuronal glutamate and GABAA receptor function in health and disease. *Biochem Soc Trans.* 2009;(37):1317-22.

Mulley JC, Sche.er IE, Petrou S, Berkovic SF. Channelopathies as a genetic cause of epilepsy. *Curr Opin Neurol.*2003;(16):171-6.

Nelson DR, Zeldin DC, Hoffman SMG, Maltais LJ, Wain HM, et al. Comparison of cytochrome P450 (CYP) genes from the mouse and human genomes, including nomenclature recommendations for genes, pseudogenes and alternative-splice variants. *Pharmacogenetics.*2004;(14): 1-18.

Ragsdale DS, McPhee JC, Scheuer T, Catterall WA. Common molecular determinants of local anesthetic, antiarrhythmic, and anticonvulsant block of voltage-gated Na+ channels. *Proc Natl Acad Sci USA.* 1996; (93):9270-5.

Reid CA, Berkovic SF, Petrou S. Mechanisms of human inherited epilepsies. *Neurobiol.*2009;(87):41-57.

Rogawski MA, Loscher W. The neurobiology of antiepileptic drugs. *Nat Rev Neurosci.* 2004;(5):553–64.

Siddiqui A, Kerb R, Weale ME, Brinkmann U, Smith A, Goldstein DB, Wood NW and Sisodiya SM. Association of multidrug resistance in epilepsy with a polymorphism in the drug-transporter gene ABCB1. *N Engl J Med.*2003;(348):1442-1448.

Sisodiya SM and Marini C. Genetics of antiepileptic drug resistance. *Current Opinion Neurol* 2009;(22):150–156.

Sisodiya SM, Lin WR, Harding BN, Squier MV and Thom M. Drug resistance in epilepsy: expression of drug resistance proteins in common causes of refractory epilepsy. *Brain.* 2002;(125):22-31.

Steijns LS, van Weelden MJ and de Haan K. The effect of genetic polymorphism of cytochrome P450 CYP2C9 on phenytoin dose requirement. *Pharmacogenetics.* 2001;(11):287-291.

Szoeke C, Sills GJ, Kwan P, Petrovski S, Newton M, Hitiris N, Baum L, Berkovic SF, Brodie MJ, Sheffield LJ and O'Brien TJ. Multidrug-resistant genotype (ABCB1) and seizure recurrence in newly treated epilepsy: Data from International Pharmacogenetic Cohorts. *Epilepsia.*2009;(50):1689-1696.

Szoeke CE, Newton M, Wood JM, Goldstein D, Berkovic SF, OBrien TJ, et al. Update on pharmacogenetics inepilepsy: A brief review. *Lancet Neurol.* 2006;(5):189-96.

Tate SK, Depondt C, Sisodiya SM, Cavalleri GL, Schorge S, Soranzo N, Thom M, Sen A, Shorvon SD, Sander JW, Wood NW, Goldstein DB. Genetic predictors of the maximum doses patients receive during clinical use of the anti-epileptic drugs carbamazepine and phenytoin. *Proc Natl Acad Sci USA.* 2005;(102):5507–12.

Tate SK, Singh R, Hung CC, Tai JJ, Depondt C, Cavalleri GL, Sisodiya SM, Goldstein DB, Liou HH. A common Sodium channel SCN1A and SCN2A in epilepsy Br polymorphism in the SCN1A gene associates with phenytoin serum levels at maintenance dose. *Pharmacogenet Genomics* 2006;(16):721–26.

Tishler DM, Weinberg KI, Hinton DR, Barbaro N, Annett GM and Raffel C. MDR1 gene expression in brain of patients with medically intractable epilepsy. *Epilepsia.*1995;(36): 1-6.

van der Weide J, Steijns L.S, van Weelden M.J. and de Haan, K. The effect of genetic polymorphism of cytochrome P450 CYP2C9 on phenytoin dose requirement. *Pharmacogenetics.*2001; (11):287-291.

Wang L, McLeod HL and Weinshilboum RM. *Genomics and Drug Response N Engl J Med* 2011;(364):1144-53.

Wilson JF, Weale ME, Smith AC, Gratrix F, Fletcher B, et al. Population genetic structure of variable drug response. *Nat Genet.*2001;29(3):265-9.

Woodcock J. Assessing the clinical utility of diagnostics used in drug therapy. *Clin Pharmacol Ther.* 2010;(88):765-73.

Xie X, Dale TJ, John VH, Cater HL, Peakman TC, Clare JJ. Electrophysiological and pharmacological properties of the human brain type IIA Na+ channel expressed in a stable mammalian cell line. *P.ugers Arch.*2001;(441):425-33.

In: Seizures and Anti-Epileptic Drugs
Editors: Willard Hosten and Aleph Burtsev
ISBN: 978-1-62100-255-0

Chapter VII

Panayiotopoulos Syndrome: Clinical, Electroencephalographic, Genetic and Neurocognitive Characteristics

Ayse Destina Yalcin[1,*] and Asli Demirtas-Tatlidede[2]
[1]Sisli Etfal Research and Training Hospital, Department of Neurology, Istanbul, Turkey
[2]Bakirkoy Sadi Konuk Research and Training Hospital,
Department of Neurology, Istanbul, Turkey

Abstract

Panayiotopoulos Syndrome is one of the benign childhood seizure susceptibility syndromes, which has drawn increasing attention in the last decade. Panayiotopoulos Syndrome is common, affecting around 6% of children with afebrile seizures, manifests as autonomic seizures and autonomic status epilepticus that are specific to childhood, provides links with mainly rolandic epilepsy, and is frequently misdiagnosed as encephalitis and other nonepileptic disorders. Interictal EEG shows in 80% of patients multifocal spikes with occipital predominance often shifting from one region to another in sequential EEG recordings of the same patient.

Prognosis with respect to seizure remission and neuropsychological development is excellent. Continuous treatment with antiepileptic drugs is usually not needed. This review focuses on the clinical and electroencephalographic features of Panayiotopoulos Syndrome with particular emphasis on genetic and neurobehavioral aspects.

* Corresponding Author: Assoc. Prof. A. Destina Yalcin, Sisli Etfal Research and Training Hospital, Department of Neurology, Sisli, Istanbul, 34337 Turkey. E-mail: destinayalcin@yahoo.com.

Overview

Panayiotopoulos syndrome (PS) is best described as early-onset benign childhood seizure susceptibility syndrome with mainly autonomic seizures and autonomic status epilepticus. An expert consensus defines Panayiotopoulos syndrome as a "benign age-related focal seizure disorder occurring in early and mid-childhood, which is characterized by seizures, often prolonged, with predominantly autonomic symptoms, and by an EEG that shows shifting and/or multiple foci, often with occipital predominance" (Ferrie et al., 2006).

Panayiotopoulos syndrome is now the formally approved term for this syndrome in the new ILAE report on classification (Berg et al., 2010), thus rightly abandoning a number of previously used descriptive synonyms such as early onset benign childhood epilepsy with occipital paroxysms, early onset benign childhood occipital epilepsy, nocturnal childhood occipital epilepsy. The reason for this is that these descriptive terms are incorrect (Covanis, 2006; Ferrie et al., 2006; Caraballo et al., 2007; Koutroumanidis, 2007; Martinovic, 2007; Panayiotopoulos et al., 2008; Michael et al., 2010; Specchio et al., 2010a, b) because: (1) Onset of seizures is mainly with autonomic symptoms, which are not occipital lobe manifestations, (2) Of occipital symptoms, only deviation of the eyes may originate from the occipital regions, but this rarely occurs at onset. Visual symptoms are exceptional and not consistent in recurrent seizures, (3) Interictal occipital spikes may never occur, (4) Magnetoencephalography may show equivalent current dipoles clustering in the frontal areas (Saitoh et al., 2007), (5) Ictal EEG has documented variable onset from the posterior or anterior regions (Beaumanoir, 1993; Oguni et al., 1999; Vigevano et al., 2000; Demirbilek and Dervent, 2004; Koutroumanidis et al., 2005; Parisi et al., 2005; Iannetti et al., 2009; Specchio et al., 2010a, b).

Panayiotopoulos Syndrome (PS) was identified by the Greek epileptologist Chrysostomos P. Panayiotopoulos through long term pivotal studies in which he described autonomic seizures and autonomic status epilepticus specific to childhood (Panayiotopoulos, 1988a, 1989a,b, 1999). These were common and mainly occurred in otherwise normal children whose prognosis in terms of seizure remission and development was excellent. Their EEG was characterised by spikes and sharp waves occurring in variable localisations. These children are now classified as having Panayiotopoulos syndrome (Ferrie et al., 2006; Koutroumanidis, 2007; Berg et al. 2010). However, there was initial scepticism and resistance to these findings, including from influential epileptologists because as explained by Ferrie and Livingston (2010):

(1) ictal vomiting had been considered as extremely rare and hither to had been mainly described in neurosurgical series of adult patients. In children, it was generally not considered as having an epileptic origin;
(2) autonomic status epilepticus was not recognised as a diagnostic entity; the proposition that it might be a common occurrence in a benign seizure disorder challenged orthodox concepts of status epilepticus;
(3) it implied that paediatricians had been failing to diagnose significant numbers of children with epilepsy, instead erroneously labeling then as having diverse non-epileptic disorders such as encephalitis, syncope, migraine, cyclic vomiting syndrome and gastroenteritis;

(4) the characteristic EEG findings suggested alternative diagnoses. Occipital spikes suggested "childhood epilepsy with occipital paroxysms" of Gastaut; multifocal spikes suggested symptomatic epilepsies with poor prognosis.

"The veracity of Panayiotopoulos's initial descriptions has, over the last two decades, been confirmed in large and long term studies from Europe, Japan and South America. The published database on which our knowledge of PS is now based includes over 800 cases; there are few epilepsy syndromes which are better characterised. What emerges are a remarkably uniform clinical picture and a diagnosis which is strikingly useful in helping predict prognosis and dictate management." (Ferrie and Livingston, 2010).

PS is one of the three major syndromes of benign childhood seizure susceptibility syndrome (BCSSS), which also comprise rolandic epilepsy, and idiopathic childhood occipital epilepsy of Gastaut (ICOE-G) (Panayiotopoulos et al., 2008). BCSSS is a common, genetically determined, mild and reversible functional derangement of the cortical maturational process (Panayiotopoulos, 1993, 2010). This unified concept is classified under age and localization related idiopathic epilepsies; the epileptic seizures and the EEG abnormalities are focal (localization related), only occur in children (age related), and physical, mental and laboratory examination other than EEG are normal (idiopathic) (Koutroumanidis, 2007). A normal child with mainly nocturnal, infrequent seizures and an EEG with disproportionately severe focal epileptogenic activity is highly suggestive of BCSSS.

Epidemiology

The seizures occur between 1-14 years of age, with an onset age varying between 3-6 years in 76%. Both sexes are equally affected though female superiority preponderance was reported in some studies (Panayiotopoulos, 2002; Lada et al., 2003; Covanis, 2006; Durá-Travé et al., 2008). The prevalence of PS is around 13% of children 3 to 6 years old with 1 or more nonfebrile seizures and 6% of the age group of 1 to 15 years (Panayiotopoulos, 2002). Autonomic status epilepticus is the more common type of nonfebrile status epilepticus in normal children (Okanishi et al., 2008).

Genetics

Mutations in *SCN1A* gene, coding for the $\alpha 1$ subunit of the neuronal sodium channel, has recently been linked to PS (Grosso et al., 2007; Livingston et al., 2009). The mutation occurs within the first of 4 S4 protein segments that form the voltage sensor of the sodium channel protein. De novo mutation of *SCN1A* gene was detected in a patient with atypical PS (Grosso et al., 2007). Familial SCN1A mutation (p.Phe218Leu) was detected in two siblings with PS, while their father with the same mutation never had a seizure (Livingston et al., 2009).

The identified mutations of the *SCN1A* gene in patients with PS suggest that *SCN1A* mutations may cause susceptibility to an idiopathic focal epilepsy phenotype. However, no such mutations were found in another couple of siblings (personal communication with C.

Panayiotopoulos) and homozygous twins (Martin del Valle et al.,2011) with typical PS and no febrile seizure precipitants.

These data indicate that SCN1A mutations when found contribute to a more severe clinical phenotype of PS (Panayiotopoulos et al., 2008). Further, clinical genetic studies reported very similar concordance rates for monozygotic and dizygotic twin pairs indicating a probable role of multifactorial aetiology (genetic or environmental factors) in determining the ultimate phenotype (Taylor et al., 2008).

Clinical Characteristics

PS is characterized by prolonged seizures with predominantly autonomic symptoms (Ferrie et al., 2006, 2007; Covanis, 2006; Koutroumanidis, 2007; Caraballo et al., 2007; Specchio et al., 2010a). Restlessness, agitation, quietness, headache or various non-painful cephalic sensations may occur at the onset of seizures.

Ictus emeticus, consisting of nausea, retching and vomiting appears in 74-82 % of the seizures, usually at the beginning (Panayiotopoulos, 1989b; Ferrie et al., 1997; Oguni et al., 1999; Kivity et al., 2000).

Other autonomic manifestations include pallor, cyanosis, mydriasis and less frequently miosis, cardiac, respiratory, thermoregulatory and intestinal motility abnormalities, hypersalivation, coughing, urinary or fecal incontinence (Panayiotopoulos, 1989b; Ferrie et al., 1997).

At the beginning of the seizure, consciousness and speech are preserved as a rule. If the seizure continues, the child slowly or suddenly becomes confused and unresponsive. A peculiar ictal symptom, named as ictal syncope by Panayiotopoulos, describes total unresponsiveness of the child followed by a fall due to loss of postural tone. This occurs in 20% of the cases and can be the sole manifestation of the seizure (Panayiotopoulos, 2001, 2002, 2004; Ferrie et al., 2006; Michael et al., 2010).

The most common motor ictal symptom is the unilateral deviation of the eyes resembling pursuit like slow movement in horizontal plane, which can be continuous or intermittent, short or prolonged (Panayiotopoulos, 2002; Ferrie et al., 2006; Ferrie and Livingston, 2010). Ictal visual symptoms occur only in 10% of the affected children and usually follow the autonomic manifestations (Yalcin et al. 1997; Panayiotopoulos, 2002; Lada et al., 2003; Caraballo et al., 2007; Ferrie and Livingston, 2010).

Some authors doubt that visual symptoms cannot be used to differentiate the PS and ICOE-G, because young children are not usually able to articulate these symptoms (Taylor et al., 2008) though most of the children with PS are able to communicate their symptoms. Half of the seizures progress to hemi- or generalised convulsions (Panayiotopoulos, 2002; Panayiotopoulos et al., 2008, Caraballo et al., 2007; Specchio et al., 2010a; Ferrie and Livingston, 2010)

Other less frequent ictal features include speech arrest, hemifacial spasms, oropharyngolaryngeal movements suggesting a maturation related continuum with rolandic epilepsy (Panayiotopoulos, 1993; Koutroumanidis, 2007).

Precipitating Factors, Frequency and Duration of the Seizures

Sleep is the most common precipitating factor in PS. Two-thirds of the affected children have seizures only during sleep, including both nocturnal sleep and daytime naps (Kivity and Lerman, 1992; Maher et al., 1995; Ferrie et al., 1997, 2006; Panayiotopoulos, 2002). Many seizures are observed during traveling, most probably because children can easily fall asleep in these circumstances and traveling itself can precipitate motion sickness to which children are peculiarly susceptible (Panayiotopoulos, 2010). Most of the children with PS have two to five seizures during the active period of their illness, while one-third of the patients experience only a single seizure. Very frequent seizures are unusual but do not exclude the diagnosis; these patients are considered to have an atypical form of the disease (Kivity and Lerman, 1992; Maher et al., 1995; Caraballo et al., 1997; Ferrie et al., 1997; Covanis, 2006; Oguni et al., 1999; Panayiotopoulos, 2010; Specchio et al., 2010a). The average duration of seizures is nine minutes (Panayiotopoulos et al., 2008; Panayiotopoulos, 2010; Michael et al., 2010). The occurrence of autonomic SE is a common and important feature of the syndrome (Panayiotopoulos, 1988a; Fejerman, 1996; Kivity and Lerman, 1992; Maher et al., 1995; Ferrie et al. 2007; Panayiotopoulos et al., 2008; Covanis and Panayiotopoulos, 2008; Capovilla et al., 2009). Approximately half of the patients may suffer from autonomic SE, which may last for more than 30 minutes to many hours (Panayiotopoulos, 2002; Ferrie et al., 2007; Panayiotopoulos et al., 2008). Peculiarly, these patients will turn to normal only after a few hours of sleep. Long-lasting autonomic SE necessitates detailed evaluation of these patients, especially when it appears for the first time (Panayiotopoulos, 2010). Convulsive SE has been reported in exceptional cases (Ferrie et al., 2006; Michael et al., 2010). The seizures are expected to cease within 1-2 years following the onset, irrespective of their length and severity.

Neurobehavioral and Cognitive Aspects

Currently, there are very few studies that specifically searched for the behavioral and cognitive aspects of PS. IQ evaluations were found to be in the normal range for the vast majority of the patients with PS while borderline to mild mental retardation was present in the remaining cases (Specchio et al., 2010a; Hirano et al., 2009). In the patients with normal IQ, all subtest values were found to be within the normal limits but a significant difference was detected in arithmetic, comprehension and picture arrangement subtests when compared with controls (Specchio et al., 2010a). A significant discrepancy in verbal vs. performance IQ scores has been identified in approximately 10% of the patients (Hirano et al., 2009). Hirano and colleagues (2009) detected neurobehavioral disorders in 32% of their patients. Atypical cases, who had more than 10 recurrent seizures, appeared to show neurobehavioral abnormalities more frequently than typical patients (Hirano et al., 2009). Concurrence with attention deficit hyperactivity disorder, learning disability, and autistic spectrum disorder was present among the atypical cases (Hirano et al., 2009). Behavioral aspects of visual function and visuoperceptual abilities in PS have recently been investigated and were found to be relatively uncommon (De Rose et al., 2010). Visual assessments showed 15% abnormal crowding acuity and 4% abnormal stereopsis. Visuoperceptual evaluations, which tested dorsal and ventral visual pathway functions via form and/or motion coherence threshold measurements, revealed abnormalities in 18%. Age at onset of seizure <5 years and EEG activation after eye closure or during sleep were the suggested to increase the risk for developing visual abnormalities (De Rose et al., 2010).

Diagnostic Tests

By definition of an idiopathic syndrome, neurologic, mental, and high resolution MRI is normal. However, because of its high prevalence, PS may incidentally occur in children with neurocognitive deficits or abnormal brain scans (Yalcin et al., 2009; Ferrie and Livingston, 2010).

Electroencephalography

Electroencephalography (EEG) is the only diagnostic test to be abnormal in PS. There is marked variability of interictal EEG findings from normal to multifocal spikes that also vary in serial EEGs. In about 90% of cases, the EEG mainly shows multifocal, high amplitude, sharp and slow wave complexes that may appear in any area, shifting from one region to another in the same or controlateral hemisphere in different EEGs of the same patient (Figure 1) (Ohtsu et al., 2003, 2008; Ferrie et al., 2006; Panayiotopoulos, 2002; Panayiotopoulos et al., 2008; Caraballo et al., 2007; Specchio et al., 2010a,b). Occipital location predominates in most published reports but epileptiform activity may occur in any area, frequently in the centrotemporal and frontal regions (Covanis et al., 2003; Ferrie et al., 2006; Koutroumanidis, 2007; Specchio et al., 2010a,b). In one-third of the patients, the occipital location may be absent. Clone-like, repetitive, multifocal spike-wave complexes are very characteristic for PS (Panayiotopoulos, 2002). The background activity is normal with the exception of postictal recordings. Sleep typically accentuates the spike abnormalities, and photosensitivity is usually absent (Panayiotopoulos, 2002; Panayiotopoulos et al., 2008). If a routine EEG is interpreted as normal, a subsequent sleep EEG should be performed (Panayiotopoulos, 2002). Brief generalized discharges, comprising slow waves intermixed with small spikes may occur 4% alone and 15% with focal spikes (Panayiotopoulos et al., 2008; Panayiotopoulos, 2010). Consistently normal EEG is rare but may occur (Specchio et al., 2010b).

A recent study, examined the spatiotemporal course of interictal spikes in PS and in particular whether seemingly independent extra-occipital spikes are truly autonomous or secondary, triggered by occipital spikes (Kokkinos et al., 2010). It was found that the patterns of spatial and temporal dynamics of the interictal spikes were not stereotypical for any brain area, including the occipital lobe. Some of the anterior and the posterior spikes remained focal or showed little spread, but others appeared to propagate to the opposite direction (occipital to frontal and vice versa). The authors concluded that in PS all cerebral locations are able to spontaneously and independently generate and propagate interictal spikes, indicating that this is a multifocal epileptic syndrome (Kokkinos et al., 2010).

Fixation-off sensitivity (FOS) refers to the forms of epilepsy, EEG abnormalities or both which are elicited by elimination of central vision or fixation (Panayiotopoulos, 1981, 1988b, 2002). FOS is not specific to an epileptic syndrome but commonly associated with idiopathic cases. The prevalence of FOS in PS has been probably overestimated (Panayiotopoulos, 2010). There is no correlation between the frequency, location, persistence of the spikes and duration, severity, frequency of seizures (Panayiotopoulos, 2010).

Magnetoencephalography (MEG) studies, documenting equivalent current dipoles not only along the parietooccipital and calcarine fissures but also along the rolandic fissure, have confirmed the multifocal nature of epileptogenecity in PS (Kanazawa et al., 2005; Saitoh et al., 2007). In their more recent study, Saitoh and colleagues evaluated age-related or duration-related MEG spike localization in 25 patients with PS (Saitoh et al., 2008). Patients with frontal spikes were significantly older than patients with spikes on rolandic, parieto-occipital, or calcarine sulci. Follow-up MEG was performed on 3 patients and demonstrated shifting localization or disappearance of MEG spikes (Saitoh et al., 2008).

Ictal video-EEG has unequivocally documented the epileptic nature of the autonomic manifestations in Panayiotopoulos syndrome (Beaumanoir, 1993; Oguni et al., 1999; Vigevano et al., 2000; Demirbilek and Dervent, 2004; Koutroumanidis et al., 2005; Parisi et al., 2005; Iannetti et al., 2009; Specchio et al., 2010 a,b). These may start long after the onset of the electrical ictal discharge and manifest with tachycardia, breathing irregularities, coughing, or emesis, which would be impossible to consider as seizure events without EEG. Other recognizable conventional seizure symptoms, such as convulsions, appear later in the ictal phase or may not appear at all. The ictal discharge is characterized by rhythmic monomorphic decelerating theta or delta activity, which is markedly different than the episodic fast activity of visual seizures of ICOE-G (Beaumanoir, 1993). The onset of the ictal discharge is usually from the posterior brain regions, but frontal onset has also been documented (Oguni et al., 1999; Koutroumanidis et al., 2005; Specchio et al., 2010 a,b).

Pathophysiology

Autonomic ictal symptoms of any type can be observed in seizures of both adults and children. These symptoms are generated by activation or inhibition of different parts of the autonomic central network, which involves insular cortex, medial prefrontal cortex, amygdala, hypothalamus, periaquaductal gray matter, parabranchial complex of the pons, nucleus of the tractus solitarius and ventrolateral medulla. It is generally accepted that autonomic seizures, especially ictus emeticus, are strongly age-related and much more common in children. On the other hand, ictal vomiting rarely occurs in adults, mainly following impairment of consciousness and other focal temporal lobe symptoms, and has been related to the non-dominant temporal lobe (Ferrie et al., 2007; Koutroumanidis, 2007; Panayiotopoulos et al., 2008; Panayiotopoulos, 2010). The ictal EEG recordings of autonomic seizures in PS revealed the evidence that the ictal vomiting may arise from different cortical regions and likely has no localizing or lateralizing value. The preferential involvement of emetic and other ictal symptoms in PS have been attributed to a maturation-related susceptibility of the central autonomic network (Panayiotopoulos 2002, 2004; Michael et al., 2010). Irrespective of the localization, the ictal discharge may first activate the autonomic centers because of their lower threshold, before it activates the other cortical regions with relatively higher threshold that generate cortical symptoms such as sensorial, motor, visual or other. Seizures may comprise merely autonomic symptoms if ictal neuronal activation of non-autonomic cortical areas fails to reach the symptomatogenic zone. Another question related to the relatively long duration of seizures in PS and the high frequency of autonomic status epilepticus (SE) is the failure of the inhibitory mechanisms that usually terminate a common seizure in a matter of few minutes (Ferrie et al., 2007; Koutroumanidis, 2007; Panayiotopoulos et al., 2008; Panayiotopoulos, 2010).

Differential Diagnosis

The clinical features of PS are frequently mistaken for nonepileptic conditions such as acute encephalitis, syncope, migraine, cyclic vomiting syndrome, motion sickness, sleep disorder or gastroenteritis (Covanis, 2006). However, the semiological sequence of autonomic ictal symptoms in PS can enable the correct diagnosis and recognition of this syndrome. On the other hand, the autonomic symptoms are relatively uncommon seizure manifestations and are frequently considered to be related to other non-epileptic events (Durá-Travé et al., 2008; Covanis and Panayiotopoulos, 2008; Panayiotopoulos, 2010). In the acute stage, clouding of consciousness followed by convulsions may indicate encephalitis or other acute cerebral insult. When cephalic auras occur at headache onset, the condition can be likely diagnosed as migraine in the absence of other autonomic symptoms (Panayiotopoulos, 2002; Ferrie et al., 2006; Ferrie and Livingston, 2010). If ictal syncope, accompanied by falling down and unresponsiveness, lasts longer, encephalitic states resulting from infection or various metabolic causes, raised intracranial pressure and others diagnoses must be excluded with appropriate investigations (Panayiotopoulos, 2002, 2010; Ferrie et al., 2006). History of a previous similar event or full recovery after few hours sleep even after autonomic SE may help to avoid unnecessary investigations and treatments. Ten to twenty percent of the children with autonomic seizures can have heterogeneous cerebral pathology and these patients may reveal abnormalities in mental and/or neurological examination, brain imaging and the EEG background (Covanis and Panayiotopoulos, 2008; Ferrie and Livingston, 2010; Panayiotopoulos, 2010).

Prognosis

PS is a remarkably benign condition as documented in long-term studies including over 1000 children worldwide even in those with coincidental brain lesions (Panayiotopoulos, 1988a, 1989b, 2002, 2010; Parisi et al. 2007; Yalcin et al., 2009). The risk of developing epilepsy in adult life is not higher than the general population, however, further studies with long-term follow-up are required to confirm this assumption (Ferrie et al., 2006; Covanis and Panayiotopoulos, 2008; Ferrie and Livingston, 2010; Michael et al., 2010). Approximately one-fifth of the children with this syndrome may later develop other types of infrequent seizures (most frequently rolandic seizures followed by visual seizures) but all these are age related and remit before the age of 16 (Ferrie et al., 2006; Panayiotopoulos, 2002, 2010). It would be convenient to keep a strict evolutional follow-up in these patients as an atypical evolution might occur (Dura-Trave et al., 2008); five atypical cases were reported to develop seizure types other than mentioned above. These patients had reversible cognitive and behavioral problems, sometimes associated with continuous spike and slow wave activity during sleep (Caraballo et al., 2001; Ferrie et al., 2002; Ferrie and Livingston, 2010). Among them, two showed an atypical course and a more severe phenotype of PS, which was demonstrated to be probably related to SCN1A mutation (Grosso et al., 2007; Livingstone et al., 2009). It must be kept in mind that autonomic seizures can be life threatening if they are associated with cardiac arrest (Panayiotopoulos, 2002; Verrotti et al., 2005; Ferrie et al., 2006).

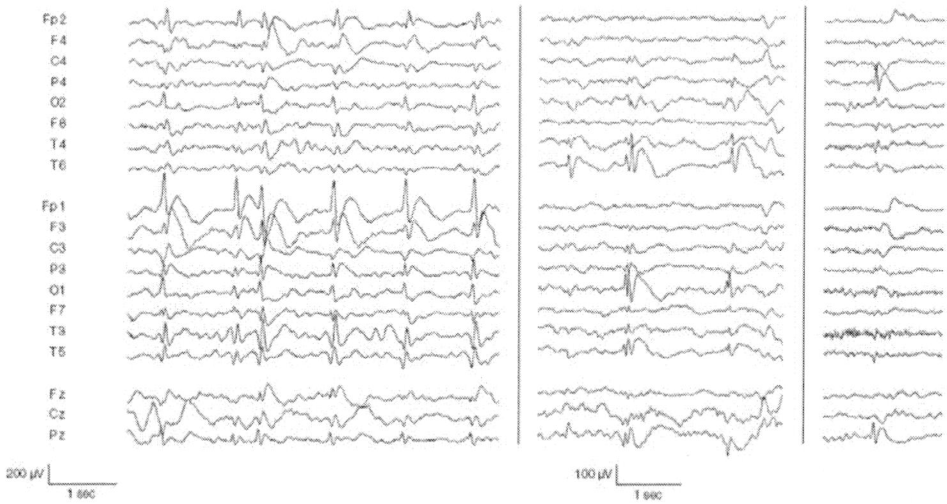

Figure 1. Interictal EEG samples of three patients with PS. Typically, high amplitude repetitive spikes occur in all locations while sometimes spike activity may be scarce with small amplitudes. Modified with permission from C. P. Panayiotopoulos (2010).

Treatment

Prophylactic antiepileptic treatment may not be needed for the majority of the patients (Ferrie et al., 2006; Covanis and Panayiotopoulos, 2008; Ferrie and Livingston; 2010). However, the education of the parents about the nature and prognosis of the syndrome is critical (Valeta, 2005). The parents need specific information about PS, in which seizures can last for many hours (Valeta, 2005; Ferrie et al., 2006; Covanis and Panayiotopoulos; 2008; Panayiotopoulos, 2010). Regular antiepileptic drug treatment in PS is recommended only for those children, in whom seizures are very frequent or are interfering with the quality of life. There is no evidence that any particular antiepileptic drug has therapeutic superiority over the others. Of the established antiepileptic drugs, carbamazepine and sodium valproate are the most frequently used ones and appear to be equally effective (Wheless and Bourgeois, 2004; Ferrie et al., 2006; Wheless and Clarke, 2007; Covanis and Panayiotopoulos, 2008). Carbamazepine has been reported to cause an exacerbation in the EEG and seizures in one case (Kikumoto et al., 2006). Our knowledge of the efficacy of the new antiepileptic drugs in PS is currently limited (Garcia and Rubio, 2009).

Acknowledgment

The authors are grateful to Dr. Chrysostomos Panayiotopoulos for reviewing this manuscript and his valuable comments.

References

Beaumanoir A (1993). Semiology of occipital seizures in infants and children. In: Andermann F, Beaumanoir A, Mira L, Roger J, Tassinari CA, editors. *Occipital seizures and epilepsies in children.* London: John Libbey and Company Ltd; 71-86.

Berg AT, Berkovic SF, Brodie MJ, Buchhalter J, Cross JH, van Emde Boas W, Engel J, French J, Glauser TA, Mathern GW, Moshé SL, Nordli D, Plouin P, Scheffer IE (2010). Revised terminology and concepts for organization of seizures and epilepsies: Report of the ILAE Commission on Classification and Terminology, 2005-2009. *Epilepsia* 51, 676-685.

Caraballo RH, Cersósimo RO, Medina CS, Tenembaum S, Fejerman N (1997). Idiopathic partial epilepsy with occipital paroxysms. *Rev Neurol.* 25, 1052-8.

Caraballo RH, Astorino F, Cersósimo R, Soprano AM, Fejerman N (2001). Atypical evolution in childhood epilepsy with occipital paroxysms (Panayiotopoulos type). *Epileptic Disord.* 3, 157-62.

Caraballo R, Cersósimo R, Fejerman N (2007). Panayiotopoulos syndrome: a prospective study of 192 patients. *Epilepsia.* 48, 1054-61.

Covanis A, Lada C, Skiadas K (2003). Children with Rolandic spikes and ictal vomiting: Rolandic epilepsy or Panayiotopoulos syndrome? *Epileptic Disord.* 5, 139-43.

Covanis A (2006). Panayiotopoulos syndrome: a benign childhood autonomic epilepsy frequently imitating encephalitis, syncope, migraine, sleep disorder, or gastroenteritis. *Pediatrics.* 118, e1237-43.

Covanis A, Panayiotopoulos CP (2008). Improving the diagnostic yield in Panayiotopoulos syndrome. *Eur J Neurol.* 15, 317-9.

De Rose P, Perrino F, Lettori D, Alfieri P, Cesarini L, Battaglia D, Ricci D, Guzzetta F, Mercuri E (2010). Visual and visuoperceptual function in children with Panayiotopoulos syndrome. *Epilepsia.* 51, 1205-11.

Demirbilek V, Dervent A (2004). Panayiotopoulos syndrome: video-EEG illustration of a typical seizure. *Epileptic Disord.* 6, 121-4.

Durá-Travé T, Yoldi-Petri ME, Gallinas-Victoriano F (2008). Panayiotopoulos syndrome: epidemiological and clinical characteristics and outcome. *Eur J Neurol.* 15, 336-41.

Fejerman N (1996). Atypical evolution of benign partial epilepsy in children. *Rev Neurol.* 24, 1415-20.

Ferrie CD, Beaumanoir A, Guerrini R, Kivity S, Vigevano F, Takaishi Y, Watanabe K, Mira L, Capizzi G, Costa P, Valseriati D, Grioni D, Lerman P, Ricci S, Vigliano P, Goumas-

Kartalas A, Hashimoto K, Robinson RO, Panayiotopoulos CP (1997). Early-onset benign occipital seizure susceptibility syndrome. *Epilepsia.* 38, 285-93.

Ferrie CD, Koutroumanidis M, Rowlinson S, Sanders S, Panayiotopoulos CP (2002). Atypical evolution of Panayiotopoulos syndrome: a case report. *Epileptic Disord.* 4, 35-42.

Ferrie C, Caraballo R, Covanis A, Demirbilek V, Dervent A, Kivity S, Koutroumanidis M, Martinovic Z, Oguni H, Verrotti A, Vigevano F, Watanabe K, Yalcin D, Yoshinaga H (2006). Panayiotopoulos syndrome: a consensus view. *Dev Med Child Neurol* 48, 236-240.

Ferrie CD, Caraballo R, Covanis A, Demirbilek V, Dervent A, Fejerman N, Fusco L, Grünewald RA, Kanazawa O, Koutroumanidis M, Lada C, Livingston JH, Nicotra A, Oguni H, Martinovic Z, Nordli DR Jr, Parisi P, Scott RC, Specchio N, Verrotti A, Vigevano F, Walker MC, Watanabe K, Yoshinaga H, Panayiotopoulos CP (2007). Autonomic status epilepticus in Panayiotopoulos syndrome and other childhood and adult epilepsies: a consensus view. *Epilepsia.* 48, 1165-72.

Ferrie CD, Livingston JH (2010). Panayiotopoulos syndrome: learning lessons from atypical cases. *Epileptic Disord.* 12, 92-4.

García C, Rubio G (2009). Efficacy and safety of levetiracetam in the treatment of Panayiotopoulos syndrome. *Epilepsy Res.* 85, 318-20.

Grosso S, Orrico A, Galli L, Di Bartolo R, Sorrentino V, Balestri P (2007). SCN1A mutation associated with atypical Panayiotopoulos syndrome. *Neurology.* 69, 609-11.

Hirano Y, Oguni H, Funatsuka M, Imai K, Osawa M (2009). Neurobehavioral abnormalities may correlate with increased seizure burden in children with Panayiotopoulos syndrome. *Pediatr Neurol.* 4, 443-8.

Iannetti P, Spalice A, Rocchi V, Verrotti A (2009). Diffuse onset of ictal electroencephalography in a typical case of Panayiotopoulos syndrome and review of the literature. *J Child Neurol* 24, 472-6.

Kanazawa O, Tohyama J, Akasaka N, Kamimura T (2005). A magnetoencephalographic study of patients with Panayiotopoulos syndrome. *Epilepsia* 46, 1106-13.

Kikumoto K, Yoshinaga H, Oka M, Ito M, Endoh F, Akiyama T, Ohtsuka Y (2006). EEG and seizure exacerbation induced by carbamazepine in Panayiotopoulos syndrome. *Epileptic Disord* 8, 53-6.

Kivity S, Lerman P (1992). Stormy onset with prolonged loss of consciousness in benign childhood epilepsy with occipital paroxysms. *J Neurol Neurosurg Psychiatry.* 55, 45-8.

Kivity S, Ephraim T, Weitz R, Tamir A (2000). Childhood epilepsy with occipital paroxysms: clinical variants in 134 patients. *Epilepsia.* 41, 1522-33.

Kokkinos V, Koutroumanidis M, Tsatsou K, Koupparis A, Tsiptsios D, Panayiotopoulos CP (2010). Multifocal spatiotemporal distribution of interictal spikes in Panayiotopoulos syndrome. *Clin Neurophysiol* 121, 859-69.

Koutroumanidis M, Rowlinson S, Sanders S (2005). Recurrent autonomic status epilepticus in Panayiotopoulos syndrome: video/EEG studies. *Epilepsy Behav.* 7, 543-7.

Koutroumanidis M (2007). Panayiotopoulos syndrome: an important electroclinical example of benign childhood system epilepsy. *Epilepsia.* 48, 1044-53.

Lada C, Skiadas K, Theodorou V, Loli N, Covanis A (2003). A study of 43 patients with panayiotopoulos syndrome, a common and benign childhood seizure susceptibility. *Epilepsia.* 44, 81-8.

Livingston JH, Cross JH, Mclellan A, Birch R, Zuberi SM (2009). A novel inherited mutation in the voltage sensor region of SCN1A is associated with Panayiotopoulos syndrome in siblings and generalized epilepsy with febrile seizures plus. *J Child Neurol.* 24, 503-8.

Maher J, Ronen GM, Ogunyemi AO, Goulden KJ (1995). Occipital paroxysmal discharges suppressed by eye opening: variability in clinical and seizure manifestations in childhood. *Epilepsia* 36, 52-7.

Martín Del Valle F, Díaz Negrillo A, Ares Mateos G, Sanz Santaeufemia FJ, Del Rosal Rabes T, González-Valcárcel Sánchez-Puelles FJ (2011). Panayiotopoulos syndrome: Probable genetic origin, but not in SCN1A. *Eur J Paediatr Neurol* 15, 155-7.

Martinovic Z (2007). The new ILAE report on classification and evidence-based commentary on Panayiotopoulos syndrome and autonomic status epilepticus. *Epilepsia* 48, 1215-6.

Michael M, Tsatsou K, Ferrie CD (2010). Panayiotopoulos syndrome: an important childhood autonomic epilepsy to be differentiated from occipital epilepsy and acute non-epileptic disorders. *Brain Dev.* 32, 4-9.

Oguni H, Hayashi K, Imai K, Hirano Y, Mutoh A, Osawa M (1999). Study on the early-onset variant of benign childhood epilepsy with occipital paroxysms otherwise described as early-onset benign occipital seizure susceptibility syndrome. *Epilepsia.* 40, 1020-30.

Ohtsu M, Oguni H, Hayashi K, Funatsuka M, Imai K, Osawa M (2003). EEG in children with early-onset benign occipital seizure susceptibility syndrome: Panayiotopoulos syndrome. *Epilepsia* 44, 435-42.

Ohtsu M, Oguni H, Imai K, Funatsuka M, Osawa M (2008). Early-onset form of benign childhood epilepsy with centro-temporal EEG foci - a different nosological perspective from Panayiotopoulos syndrome. *Neuropediatrics* 39, 14-9.

Okanishi T, Maegaki Y, Ohno K, Togari H (2008). Underlying neurologic disorders and recurrence rates of status epilepticus in childhood. *Brain Dev* 30, 624-8.

Panayiotopoulos CP (1981). Inhibitory effect of central vision on occipital lobe seizures. *Neurology.* 31, 1330-3.

Panayiotopoulos CP (1988a). Vomiting as an ictal manifestation of epileptic seizures and syndromes. *J Neurol Neurosurg Psychiatry.* 51, 1448-51.

Panayiotopoulos CP (1988b). Fixation-off, scotosensitive and other visual-related epilepsies. *Adv Neurol* 75, 139-57.

Panayiotopoulos CP (1989a). Benign nocturnal childhood occipital epilepsy: a new syndrome with nocturnal seizures, tonic deviation of the eyes, and vomiting. *J Child Neurol.* 4:43-9.

Panayiotopoulos CP (1989b). Benign childhood epilepsy with occipital paroxysms: a 15-year prospective study. *Ann Neurol.* 26:51-6.

Panayiotopoulos CP (1993). Benign childhood partial epilepsies: benign childhood seizure susceptibility syndromes. *J Neurol Neurosurg Psychiatry.* 56, 2-5.

Panayiotopoulos CP (1999) Extraoccipital benign childhood partial seizures with ictal vomiting and excellent prognosis. *J Neurol Neurosurg Psychiatry* 66, 82-85.

Panayiotopoulos CP (2002). *Panayiotopoulos Syndrome: a common and benign childhood epileptic syndrome.* London: John Libbey and Co. Ltd.

Panayiotopoulos CP (2004). Autonomic seizures and autonomic status epilepticus peculiar to childhood: diagnosis and management. *Epilepsy Behav.* 5, 286-95.

Panayiotopoulos CP, Michael M, Sanders S, Valeta T, Koutroumanidis M (2008). Benign childhood focal epilepsies: assessment of established and newly recognized syndromes. *Brain.* 131, 2264-86.

Panayiotopoulos CP (2010). Benign childhood focal seizures and related epileptic syndromes. In: *A clinical guide to epileptic syndromes and their treatment*. Revised second edition. London: Springer Healthcare Ltd.; 339-75.

Parisi P, Ferri R, Pagani J, Cecili M, Montemitro E, Villa MP (2005). Ictal video-polysomnography and EEG spectral analysis in a child with severe Panayiotopoulos syndrome. *Epileptic Disord.* 7, 333-9.

Parisi P, Villa MP, Pelliccia A, Rollo VC, Chiarelli F, Verrotti A (2007). Panayiotopoulos syndrome: diagnosis and management. *Neurol Sci.* 28, 72-9.

Saitoh N, Kanazawa O, Tohyama J, Akasaka N, Kamimura T (2007). Magnetoencephalographic findings of Panayiotopoulos syndrome with frontal epileptic discharges. *Pediatr Neurol.* 36, 190-4.

Saitoh N, Kanazawa O, Tohyama J, Akasaka N, Kamimura T, Toyabe S, Uchiyama M (2008). Brain maturation-related spike localization in Panayiotopoulos syndrome: magnetoencephalographic study. *Pediatr Neurol* 38, 104-10.

Specchio N, Trivisano M, Di Ciommo V, Cappelletti S, Masciarelli G, Volkov J, Fusco L, Vigevano F (2010a). Panayiotopoulos syndrome: a clinical, EEG, and neuropsychological study of 93 consecutive patients. *Epilepsia.* 51, 2098-107.

Specchio N, Trivisano M, Claps D, Battaglia D, Fusco L and Vigevano F (2010b). Documentation of autonomic seizures and autonomic status epilepticus with ictal EEG in Panayiotopoulos syndrome. *Epilepsy Behav* 19, 383-393.

Taylor I, Berkovic SF, Kivity S, Scheffer IE (2008). Benign occipital epilepsies of childhood: clinical features and genetics. *Brain.* 131, 2287-94.

Valeta T (2005). Parental attitude, reaction and education in benign childhood focal seizures. In: Panayiotopoulos CP, editor. *The epilepsies: seizures, syndromes and management.* Oxford: Bladon Medical Publishing; 258-61.

Verrotti A, Salladini C, Trotta D, di Corcia G, Chiarelli F (2005). Ictal cardiorespiratory arrest in Panayiotopoulos syndrome. *Neurology.* 64, 1816-7.

Vigevano F, Lispi ML, Ricci S (2000). Early onset benign occipital susceptibility syndrome: video-EEG documentation of an illustrative case. *Clin Neurophysiol.* 111 Suppl 2, S81-6.

Wheless JW, Bourgeois BF (2004). Choosing antiepileptic drugs for developmentally normal children with specific epilepsy syndromes and behavioral disorders. *J Child Neurol.* 19 Suppl 1, S39-48.

Wheless JW, Clarke DF, Arzimanoglou A, Carpenter D (2007). Treatment of pediatric epilepsy: European expert opinion, 2007. *Epileptic Disord.* 9, 353-412.

Yalcin AD, Kaymaz A, Forta H (1997) . Childhood occipital epilepsy: seizure manifestations and electroencephalographic features. *Brain Dev* 9, 408-13.

Yalcin AD, Toydemir HE, Celebi LG, Forta H (2009). Panayiotopoulos syndrome with coincidental brain lesions. *Epileptic Disord.* 11, 270-6.

Reviewed by Chrysostomos P. Panayiotopoulos, MD, PhD, FRCP

Department of Clinical Neurophysiology and Epilepsies, St Thomas' Hospital, London, and Locum Consultant Neurologist, John Radcliffe Hospital, Oxford, UK.

In: Seizures and Anti-Epileptic Drugs
Editors: Willard Hosten and Aleph Burtsev
ISBN: 978-1-62100-255-0

Chapter VIII

Behavioral Profiles of Anti-Epileptic Drugs in Patients with Epilepsy

Andrea Eugenio Cavanna[1,2,*] and Fizzah Ali[2]
[1,2]Institute of Neurology, UCL, London, United Kingdom
[2]Department of Neuropsychiatry, University of Birmingham and BSMHFT, Birmingham, United Kingdom

Abstract

Epilepsy affects different domains of an individual's life: in addition to health, independence, education and employment are all tainted. Beyond seizures, changes in mental health, behavioral alterations and variable cognitive function are central to epilepsy. Several studies have explored the relationship between behavioral impairment and seizure-related variables. In more recent years, particular emphasis has been placed on the clinical challenge presented by anti-epileptic drugs (AEDs). AEDs have various mechanisms of action and therefore generate a wide and diverse spectrum of anti-convulsant, psychiatric, and adverse effect profiles. AEDs may be presented in two classes, divided according to predominant psychotropic profile. The first group consists of valproate, gabapentin, tiagabine and vigabatrin. This cluster is characterized by potentiation of gamma-aminobutyric acid inhibitory neurotransmission. Resultant effects include cognitive slowing, anxiolytic as well anti-manic effects. Conversely, a second cluster is defined by predominantly glutamate excitatory neurotransmission. This cluster includes lamotrigine and felbamate, and is associated with activating and anti-depressant effects. In accordance with this dual classification system, the present chapter provides a detailed description of the behavioral profile of the newer AEDs. Additionally, a brief discussion on aspects such as clinical indications, pharmacology, toxicology, efficacy and tolerability is included. It is essential that AEDs therapy offers an acceptable balance between optimum seizure control and minimal disturbance to behavior and cognition.

---

[*] Correspondence: Dr Andrea E. Cavanna MD PhD. Department of Neuropsychiatry, University of Birmingham and BSMHFT, Barberry Building, 25 Vincent Drive, B152TT Birmingham, United Kingdom. Email: a.cavanna@ion.ucl.ac.uk

Keywords: Antiepileptic drugs; epilepsy; behaviour; adverse effects

1. Introduction

1.1. Treating Epilepsy: A Transformation over Ages

Understanding of epileptic aetiology has steadily metamorphosed from primitive spiritual deductions through to complex neurobiological networks. In ancient times epilepsy was proclaimed to be the 'Sacred Disease'; a product of supernatural activity ranging demonic possession, celestial influence and the natural influences of predisposing humours. As the medical understanding of epileptic aetiology has transformed over the ages, so in parallel has therapeutic mainstay evolved.

Reinstatement of humours and exorcisms have given way to evidence-based pharmacological agents. Consistent over time, however, is the immense burden epilepsy imposes on the lives of sufferers. The impact of epilepsy can only in part be attributed to the presence of physical seizure activity.

Life domains such as education and employment, social functioning and social life are all implicated [1,2]. Furthermore, previous studies have indicated the more frequent occurrence of cognitive and behavioral effects in epilepsy compared to other chronic diseases [3]. Seizure frequency, disease duration and anti-epileptic medication (AEDs) are some of the most important clinical factors affecting quality of life in epilepsy [4,5,6,7].

1.2. Introducing Anti-epileptic Drugs

Typically AED treatment is required over long time periods; from several years through to life-long treatment. Over such time periods a variety of AED induced side-effects may present. Some effects occur on initiation of therapy; these immediate effects may be considered benign because of the development of habituation [8], and other effects are reversible on dose reduction.

Conversely, there are those chronic effects that have an insidious onset and become apparent after longer periods of treatment [9]. These effects tend not to be dose-related and may involve the metabolic, endocrine, musculoskeletal and nervous systems [10,11].

Within the nervous system the vast repertoire of effects range from neurotoxicity through to cognitive consequences.

The principle focus of this chapter is a sub-group of chronic effects involving the central nervous system - the behavioral effects of AEDs. The majority of AED are deemed to have mood-modulating effects and play a role in the treatment of numerous affective disorders, particularly bipolar disorders [12]. These mood-modulating profiles of AEDs may be divided in two classes.

This chapter commences with a brief discussion on the psychiatric profile of epilepsy, with the larger part of discussion focusing on the behavioral expressions of AEDs.

2. A Brief History of Anti-Epileptic Medication

Phenytoin, carbamazepine, valproate, phenobarbitol and benzodiazepines comprise a group of 'traditional' AEDs. Use of older agents is limited as a result of pharmokinetic disadvantages and potential teratogenicity; newer agents display better seizure control and lower risk of side-effects. Use of older agents is further limited as a result of adverse impacts on cognitive profile leading to impairment in quality of life. Moreover 20-30% of patients are refractory to these drugs [13]. Eleven new drugs have since become available: (in chronological order): felbamate, vigabatrin, lamotrigine, gabapentin, topiramate, tiagabine, oxcar- bazepine, levetiracetam, zonisamide, eslicarbazepine, and lacosamide [14].

2.1. Psychopathology in Epilepsy

A mixture of neurobiological and psychosocial factors contribute to psychopathology in epilepsy, AEDs comprise only one of the contributing factors. The triad of a patients biological and psychological inclinations, the specific psychotropic influences of an individual drug as well as the intrinsic impact of epilepsy wholly contribute to effects on mood and behavior.

Compared to other chronic disorders patients with epilepsy have higher rates of mood disorders [15,16]. Mood disorders have a prevalence of 20-50% in patients with epilepsy, and feature as the most common psychiatric co-morbidity [17].

Individuals with poorly controlled epilepsy are cited as having greater prevalence of epilepsy [18]. An estimated 30% to 70% of patients with epilepsy are affected by a depressive disorder in their lifetime. [19] The presentation of depression in patients with epilepsy may be atypical [16, 20].

Alternatively, an affective disorder characterized by eight cardinal symptoms has been described [16, 21]. 'Labile depressive symptoms' (depressive mood, anergia, insomnia, pain), 'labile affective symptoms' (anxiety, fear) and 'specific symptoms' (euphoric mood, paroxysmal irritability) comprise this atypical entity, preferentially termed 'dysthymia-like disorder of epilepsy' [16, 18]. Hippocrates perceived that patients with epilepsy were likely to develop depression and vice versa [17].

More recently it has been noted that people with depression have a three to seven times greater risk of developing epilepsy [17, 22]. Aside from depression, anxiety disorders, psychoses and pseudoseizures also have greater prevalence in epilepsy compared to the general population [23, 24]. Both clinicians and patients face difficulty when attributing the cause of psychopathology on a background of epilepsy, to either the manifestations of AED therapy or alternatively patient related variables. In particular, the frequency of adverse behavioral effects related to AED use is complicated to ascertain due to failure to identify subtle effects and inability to recognize delayed expressions [23].

In patients developing psychoses, 40% succeeded an alteration in AED regime [25]. Those individuals with seizures difficult to control, are particularly vulnerable to psychopathology secondary to AED treatment [23].

3. Psychotropic Effects of AEDs

Standardized and clearly delineated criteria for the identification of psychotropic effects are not available. Alternatively, reported effects have been inserted into non-specific overlapping categories; affective syndromes, behavior or personality disorders, psychoses and encephalopathies [23]. Although the association between AEDs and psychopathology has been long known, for instance as with the bromides, with regards to older agents our knowledge stems largely from case series or anecdotal accounts rather than systematic data. Amidst the classical AEDs, phenobarbitol is regarded as having the most potential to generate behavioral toxicity [26]. Phenytoin has been linked to both schizophrenia-like psychoses [27] and a chronic encephalopathy [28]. Likewise, barbiturate treatment in both adults and paediatric populations has been linked to depression [29, 30]. The notion that further older agents such as carbamazepine and valproic acid have psychotropic properties has triggered the re-evaluation of AEDs from a behavioral perspective.

AEDs have measurable, albeit incompletely understood, actions on neuronal membrane and synaptic function. These actions may be summarized as involving alterations in the equilibrium between neuronal excitation and inhibition [16,31]. Two basic mechanisms of action are 1) potentiation of the gamma-aminobutyric acid (GAMA) mediated inhibitory system and 2) attenuation of excitatory glutamate neurotransmission. The psychotropic profile of anti-epileptic medication may be accordingly divided into two classes; negative and positive [32].

The first group is characterized by 'sedating' mood effects, which are employed for their resultant anxiolytic and anti-manic effects, useful in the management of conditions such as agitation. Cognitive slowing and fatigue are the predominant side-effects. The latter group generate 'activating' effects, and are used in the treatment of disorders such as hypersomnia and depression. Side-effects include hyperirritability and hyperactivity.

3.1. Negative Effects of AEDs on Mood

The concurrence of depression in patients with epilepsy can have a significant impact on quality of life, even greater than that of seizure frequency [33]. Aside from enhanced GABA neurotransmission, factors such as combination therapy, folate deficiency, forced normalization, as well as the presence of a past history of affective disorders have been associated with depressive symptoms occurring in conjunction to AED therapy [34]. Another factor implicated in AED induced depression includes small hippocampal volume [35]. Individuals with temporal lobe epilepsy (TLE) and hippocampal sclerosis have a greater likelihood of developing depression than subjects with TLE and a normal MRI scan [36]. A number of newer AEDs, including vigabatrin, tiagabine and topiramate, have been associated with depression as an adverse effect secondary to treatment. Although the use of vigabatrin is now limited as a result of concentric visual field defects that may occur, it still remains the choice of drug for infantile spasms. However, in clinical trials it has been associated with depression and other behavior disorders including agitation and psychoses [37]. Depression as a treatment emergent effect of vigabatrin tends to be associated with a past history of depression, and psychosis in those patients with more severe forms of epilepsy and those individuals developing an affective disorder [37].

Topiramate has approval for the management of epilepsy in both adult and pediatric populations, and is also used for the treatment of migraine headaches [38]. Topiramate is regarded as an AED with a mixed neurobiological profile, although its GABAergic properties are likely to predominate. Common side-effects include somnolence and psychomotor slowing [39]. Depression is one of the chief psychiatric adverse effects [40]. Associations include psychiatric history, seizure frequency and the presence of tonic-atonic seizures. Conversely, the use of recommended lower initiating doses, escalation rates and target doses are negatively associated with development of depression [41]. Tiagabine is presently infrequently used in both Europe and the United States [38]. The specific limitation of tiagabine is its paradoxical propensity to generate de novo nonconvulsive status epilepticus, as a result of a narrow therapeutic index [42]. Although the data for tiagabine is limited, it has been noted as one of the GABAergic agents connected with depressive symptoms [43]. Whereas vigabatrin and topiramate are more closely related to the development of depressive symptoms, featuring in up to 10% of patients, tiagabine proposes an intermediate prevalence of depression of about 4%. Other AEDs, such as lamotrigine, are connected with much lower rates of depression and are alternatively associated with positive effects on mood [34].

3.2. Positive Effects of AEDs on Mood

AEDs are also used in the treatment of psychiatric disorders; the positive psychotropic properties of AEDs such as carbamazepine and valproate are well recognized [44]. Some AEDs have mood stabilizing effects and display particular use in the treatment of bipolar disorder. Carbamazepine, for instance, has been item to a number of controlled studies evaluating the efficacy of this drug in acute mania against placebo, lithium and neuroleptics. It has been found to be equivalent to lithium in many cases, demonstrating anti-manic efficacy and a likely long-term mood-stabilising effect in many patients with bipolar disorder including those refractory to lithium [45]. The use of valproate in acute mania is well supported, although it has also been employed for use in both manic and depressive, as well as in the maintenance of bipolar disorder [45].

Lamotrogine is now widely used in the treatment of bipolar mood disorders. Its proposed mechanism of action involves the inhibition of voltage-sensitive sodium channels, thereby stabilizing neuronal membranes and modulating presynaptic transmitter release of excitatory amino acids such as glutamate and aspartate. The broader spectrum of anti-epileptic action in comparison to other AEDs which function on a similar mode, hints at additional mechanisms of action [46]. Evidence points to the use of lamotrigine in most seizure types including primary generalised tonic-clonic seizures and absence seizures [47]. A second mechanism involving calcium channels has additionally been proposed [48]. Lamotrigine displays anti-depressant effects in patients with bipolar and rapid cycling affective disorders [49, 50].

Levetiracetam, is approved for the adjunctive treatment of partial seizures in both adults and children. More recently it has also been approved as adjunctive therapy in the treatment of myoclonic seizures in adult and adolescent with juvenile myoclonic epilepsy. It may also be used for the treatment of partial onset seizures with or without secondary generalization [46]. Levitiracetam is found to be well tolerated and safe for patients with seizure, anxiety and cognitive disorders [51]. Some studies involving levitiracetam have shown improvement in mania scores of patients with bipolar spectrum disorders. Other work has conversely indicated a predisposition to promoting depressive and anxiety symptoms [52].

Worldwide, the principal approved clinical indication for the use of gabapentin is in neuropathic pain (diabetic or post-herpetic) [46]. However, its unapproved uses extend to a spectrum of neurological and psychiatric conditions [53]. Placebo –controlled trials have demonstrated the efficacy of Pregabalin in patients with partial seizures with and without secondary generalization, in neuropathic pain and generalized anxiety disorder [54, 55, 56]. It has also shown positive effects in insomnia [57].

There are other new AEDs which have not demonstrated any efficacy in primary psychiatric disorders. For instance, tiagabine has generated mostly negative results [58], and topiramate has failed to demonstrate consistent benefit in affective disorders.

4. Psychoses and Behavioral Changes

AED therapy has also been linked to the development of psychosis. Amongst patients who developed major depression or a schizophreniform psychosis, 15% of psychotic episodes were ascribed to AED treatment, including instances of forced normalization [59]. The concept of forced normalization (FN), whereby an improved EEG appearance is associated with worse psychosis, is noted as one of the possible causes [60]

Its clinical sister, alternative psychosis, refers to the pairing of well-controlled seizures to worsening psychosis. Both states have been associated with the classic and newer agents, but are especially common with the more potent AEDs, for example vigabatrin and topiramate. [23] Psychosis has been additionally been described in association with felbamate [61], tiagabine [62], zonisamide [63] and levetiracetam [64]. Moreover, case reports suggest the possible connection between lamotrigine and psychosis.

Psychoses reported in relation to newer agents tends to have been evidenced by early clinical trials. Both rapid dosing schedules or high doses, as well as the scrutiny of difficult-to-treat populations with epilepsy or patients with temporal lobe epilepsy were implicated in such trials. Although particular AED agents are more strongly associated with psychosis, this adverse state tends to occur in those susceptible to developing psychopathology [32].

Despite claims implicating social stigma and neurological factors such as perinatal disturbances or a temporal lobe organic brain syndrome, AEDs also play a crucial part in a wide array of behavioral changes in epilepsy [32].

A conduct disorder may be precipitated in children by numerous agents, most commonly the barbiturates [59]. GABAergic medications such as vigabatrin have too been associated with similar effects; excitation, hyperkinesias and aggressive behavior, which are particularly prominent in pediatric populations with learning disabilities [41].

Levetiracetam has also been associated with aggressive behavior as well as irritability, which occurs in approximately 5% of patients [66]. Possible biological vulnerability, as well as a history of psychiatric conditions, febrile convulsions and status epilepticus are related to development of such behavioral effects [67].

Conclusion

Non-specific behavioral issues are the most frequently reported AED related psychiatric adverse effects. Depression is the most common specific diagnosis, whereas psychosis is reported notably less frequently [32]. Risk of development of such effects may be related to high doses of AEDs, rapid titration, use of multiple agents and also the severity of epilepsy [59]. Certain individuals are at greater risk of developing adverse psychiatric effects, including those with a past psychiatric history, familial predisposition and temorolimbic epilepsy [32].

Selection of an AED should commence with consideration of the seizure and epileptic syndrome to be treated. Second, the most optimal agent must be chosen for an individual patient in view of its behavioural side-effect profiles. Knowledge of culprit agents and their side-effect profile teemed with the exercise of appropriate clinical caution, including low initiating doses and slow escalation with close monitoring of predisposed individuals, should reduce the risk of adverse effects [32] and even permit clinicians to harness the psychotropic potential of AEDs for positive patient gain.

References

[1] Bishop M, Allen CA. The impact of epilepsy on quality of life: a qualitative analysis. *Epilepsy Behav 2003*;4:226–33.

[2] Thompson P, Oxley J. Social aspects of epilepsy. In: Laidlaw J, Richens A, Chadwick D, editors. *A textbook of epilepsy.* London: Churchill Livingstone; 1993. p. 661–704.

[3] Hermann BP, Vickrey B, Hays RD, et al. A comparison of health-related quality of life in patients with epilepsy, diabetes and multiple sclerosis. *Epilepsy Res* 1996;25:113–8.

[4] Djibuti M, Shakarishvili R. Influence of clinical, demographic, and socioeco- nomic variables on quality of life in patients with epilepsy: findings from Georgian study. J *Neurol Neurosurg Psychiatry* 2003;74:570–3.

[5] Senol V, Soyuer F, Arman F, Ozturk A. Influence of fatigue, depression, and demographic, socioeconomic, and clinical variables on quality of life of patients with epilepsy. *Epilepsy Behav* 2007;10:96–104.

[6] Baker GA. Assessment of quality of life in people with epilepsy: some practical implications. *Epilepsia* 2001;42(Suppl. 3):66–9.

[7] Mrabet H, Mrabet A, Zouari B, Ghachem R. Health-related quality of life of people with epilepsy compared with a general reference population: a Tunisian study. *Epilepsia* 2004;45:838–43.

[8] Kulig B, Meinardi H. Effects of antiepileptic drugs on motor activity and learned behavior in the rat. In: Meinardi H, Rowan AJ, editors. *Advances in epileptology.* Amsterdam: Swets and Zeitlinger; 1997.p. 98-104.

[9] Collaborative Group for Epidemiology of Epilepsy. Adverse reactions to antiepileptic drugs: a follow-up study of 355 patients with chronic antiepileptic drug treatment. *Epilepsia* 1988;29:787-93.

[10] Aldenkamp AP, De Krom M, Rejis R. Newer antiepileptic drugs and cognitive issues. *Epilepsia* 2003;44:21-9.

[11] Rejis R, Aldenkamp AP, De Krom M. Mood effects of anti-epileptic drugs. *Epilepsy and Behavior* 2004;5:66-76.

[12] Ketter TA, Post RM, Theodore WH. Positive and negative psychiatric effects of antiepileptic drugs in patients with seizure disorders. *Neurology* 1999;53:53-67.

[13] Beghi E. Efficacy and tolerability of the new anti-epileptic drugs: conparison of two recent guidelines. *The Lancet Neurology* 2004;3:618-21.

[14] McCabe PH. New anti-epileptic drugs for the 21st centu- ry. *Expert Opin Pharmacother* 1:633-74, 2000.

[15] Blum D, Reed M, Metz A: Prevalence of major affective disorders and manic/hypomanic symptoms in persons with epilepsy: a community survey. In: *American Academy of Neurology,* Denver, CO, USA, 2002.

[16] Dudra-Jastrzebska M, Andres-Mach MM, Luszczki JJ, Czuczwar SJ. Mood disorders in patients with epilepsy. *Pharmacological Reports* 2007;59:369-378.

[17] Kanner AM. Epilepsy and mood disorders. *Epilepsia* 2007;48:20-22.

[18] Kanner AM. Depression in epilepsy: prevalence, clinical semiology, pathogenic mechanisms and treatment. *Biol Psychiatry* 2003;54:388-98.

[19] Prueter C, Norra C: Mood disorders and their treatment in patients with epilepsy. J *Neuropsychiatry Clin Neurosci* 2005:17:20-28.

[20] Mendez MF, Cummings JL, Benson DF. Depression in epilepsy: significance and phenomenology. *Arch Neurol* 1986:43:766-770.

[21] Blumer D, Altshuler LL. Affective disorders. In: *Epilepsy: A Comprehensive Textbook.* Ed. Engel J, Pedley TA. Lippincott Raven, Philadelphia. 1998, 2083-2099.

[22] Hesdorffer DC, Hauser WA, Annegers JF, Cascino G. Makor depression is a risk factor for seizures in older adults. *Annals of Neurology* 2000;47:246-249.

[23] Schmitz B. Effects of anti-epileptic drugs on mood and behavior. *Epilepsia* 2006;47:28—33.

[24] Schmitz B, Wolf P. Psychosis with epilepsy: frequency and risk factors. J Epilepsy 1995;8:295-305.

[25] Matsuura M. Epileptic psychoses and anti-convulsant drug treatment. *J Neurol Neurosurg Psychiatry* 1999;67:231-3.

[26] Kwan P, Brodie MJ. Neuropsychological effects of epilepsy and antiepileptic drugs. *Lancet* 2001;357:216-222.

[27] McDanal CE, Bolman WM. Delayed idiosyncratic psychosis with diphenylhydantoin. *JAMA* 1975;231:1063.

[28] Trimble MR, Reynolds EH. Anticonvulsant drugs and mental symptoms: a review. *Psychol Med* 1976;6:169-78.

[29] Robertson MM, Trimble MR, Townsend HRA. Phenomenology of depression in epilepsy. *Epilepsia* 1987;28:364-72.

[30] Brent DA, Crumrine PK, Varma RR, et al. Phenobarbital treatment and major depressive disorder in children with epilepsy. *Paediatrics* 1987;80:909-17.

[31] White HS. Comparative anticonvulsant and mechanistic profile of the established and newer antiepileptic drugs. *Epilepsia* 1999;40:2-10.

[32] Mula M, Monaco F. Antiepileptic drugs and psychopathology of epilepsy: an update. *Epileptic Disord* 2009;11:1-9.

[33] Gilliam F. The impact of epilepsy on subjective health status. *Curr Neurol Neurosci Rep* 2003;3:357-62.

[34] Mula M, Sander JW. Negative effects of antiepileptic drugs on mood in patients with epilepsy. *Drug Saf* 2007;30:555-67.

[35] Quiske A, Helmstaedter C, Lux S, Elger CE. Depression in patients with temporal lobe epilepsy is related to mesial temporal sclerosis. *Epilepsy Res* 2000;39:121-5.

[36] Mula M, Trimble SR, Sander JW. The role of hippocampal sclerosis in topiramate-related depression and cognitive deficits in people with epilepsy. *Epilepsia* 2003;44:1573-7.

[37] Thomas L, Trimble M, Schmitz B, Ring H. Vigabatrin and behaviour disorders: a retrospective survey. *Epilepsy Res* 1996;25:21-7.

[38] LaRoche SM, Helmers SL. The new anti-epileptic drugs: clinical applications. *JAMA* 2004;291:615-620.

[39] Singh T. Topiramate and psychosis. *Psychiatry.* 2006;3:10-7.

[40] Mula M, Trimble MR, Lhatoo SD, Sander JW. Topiramate and psychiatric adverse events in patients with epilepsy. *Epilepsia* 2003;44:659-63.

[41] Besag FM. Behavioural effects of newer antiepileptic drugs: an update. *Expert Opin Drug Saf* 2004;3:1-8.

[42] Kellinghaus C, Dziewas R, Ludemann P. Tiagabine-related non-convulsive status epilepticus in partial epilepsy: three case reports and a review of the literature. *Seizure* 2002;11:243-249.

[43] Miller JM, Kustra RP, Vuong A, Hammer AE, Messenheimer JA. Depressive symptoms in epilepsy: prevalence, impact, aetiology, biological correlatesand effect of treatment with antiepileptic drugs. *Drugs* 2008;68:1493-509.

[44] Walden J, Normann C, Langosch J, Berger M, Grunze H. Differential treatment of bipolar disorder with old and new anti-epileptic drugs. *Neuropsychobiology* 1998;38:181-

[45] Spina E, Perugi G. Antiepileptic drugs: indications other than epilepsy. *Epileptic Disord* 2004;6:57-75.

[46] Bialer M, Johannessen SI, Kupferberg HJ, et al. Progress report on new antiepileptic drugs: a summary of the eighth Eilat Conference (EILAT VIII). *Epilepsy Research* 2007;73:1-52.

[47] Biton V, Sackellares JC, Vuong I, et al. Double-blind, placebo-controlled study of lamotrigine in primary generalized tonic-clonic seizures. *Neurology* 2005;65: 1737-1743.

[48] Stefani A, Spadoni F, Siniscalchi A, Bernardi G. Lamotrigine inhibits Ca2+ currents in cortical neurons: functional implications. *Eur J Pharmacol* 2006;307:113-116.

[49] Calabrese J, Bowden C, Sachs G, et al. A double blind placebo controlled study of lamotrigine monotherapy in outpatients with bipolar 1 depression. *J Clin Psychiatry* 1999;60:79-88.

[50] Kasumakar V, Yatham LN. An open study of lamotrigine in refractory bipolar depression. *Psychiatry Res* 1997;19:565-72.

[51] French J, Edrich P, Cramer JA. A systematic review of the safety profile of levetiracetam: a new antiepileptic drug. *Epilepsy Research* 2001;47:77-90.

[52] Gates JR, Folland C, Ankenbauer JL, Moriarty GL, Penovich PE. Behavioral side-effects of levetiracetam [abstract]. *Epilepsia* 2002;43:187.

[53] Letterman L, Markowitz JS. Gabapentin: a review of published experience in the treatment of bipolar disorder and other psychiatric conditions. *Pharmacotherapy* 1999;19:565-72.
[54] Beydoun A, Uthman BM, Kugler AR, et al. Safety and efficacy of two pregabalin regimens for add-on treatment of partial epilepsy. *Neurology* 2005;64:475-480.
[55] Arroyo S, Anhut H, Kugler AR, et al. Pregabalin add-on treatment: a randomized, double-blind, placebo controlled, dose-response study in adults with partial seizures. *Epilepsia* 2004;45:20-27.
[56] Dworkin RH, Corbin AE, Young Jr. JP, et al. Pregabalin for the treatment of postherpetic neuralgia: a randomized, placebo-controlled trial. *Neurology* 2003; 60:1274-1283.
[57] Pande AC, Crockatt JG, Feltner DE, et al. Pregabalin in generalized anxiety disorder: a placebo-controlled trial. *Am J Psychiatry* 2003;160:533-40.
[58] Grunze H, Erfuth A, Marcuse A, et al. Tiagabine appears not to be efficacious in the treatment of acute mania. *J Clin Psychiatry 1999*;13:194-9.
[59] Schmitz B. Psychiatric syndromes related to antiepileptic drugs. *Epilepsia* 1999;40: 65-70.
[60] Krishnamoorthy ES, Trimble MR. Forced normalization: clinical and therapeutic relevance. *Epilepsia* 1999;40:57-64.
[61] McConnell H, Snyder PJ, Duffy JD, et al. Neuropsychiatric side effects related to treatment with felbamate. *J Neuropsychiatry Clin Neurosci* 1996;8:341-6.
[62] Trimble MR, Rusch N, Betts T, et al. Psychiatric symptoms after therapy with new antiepileptic drugs: psychopathological and seizure-related variables. *Seizures* 2000;9:249-54.
[63] Kimura S. Zonisamide-induced behavior disorder in two children. *Epilepsia* 1994;35:403-5.
[64] Krishnamoorthy ES, Trimble MR, Sander JW, et al. Forced normalization at the interface between epilepsy and psychiatry. *Epilepsy Behav* 2002;3:303-8.
[65] Brandt C, Fueratsch N, Boehme V, et al. Development of psychosis in patients with epilepsy treated with lamotrigine: report of six cases and review of the literature. *Epilepsy Behav* 2007;11:133-9.
[66] White JR, Walczak TS, Leppik J et al. Discontinuation of levetiracetam because of behavioral side effects: a case control. *Neurology* 2003;61:1218-21.
[67] Mula M, Trimble MR, Yuen A, et al. Psychiatric adverse events during levetiracetam therapy. *Neurology* 2003;61:704-6.

In: Seizures and Anti-Epileptic Drugs
Editors: Willard Hosten and Aleph Burtsev
ISBN: 978-1-62100-255-0

Chapter IX

Addressing the Psychosocial Consequences for People Living with Seizures

Jordan Kamel and Mark Cook
St. Vincent's Hospital Melbourne, Australia

Introduction

The consequences that seizures may have on a patient's psychological and social well-being are often underestimated. People with epilepsy have much higher rates of co-morbid depression, as well as suicide, compared with the background population. Screening for depressive symptoms, as well appropriate treatment and referral, is an essential part in the management of the patient with seizures.

Although a person living with epilepsy may only spend a few minutes each year in seizure, it is the unpredictability of the next event that may necessitate lifestyle changes. It is important, however, to balance the risks of subsequent seizures with the psychosocial implications of placing restrictions on the patient's work and lifestyle.

This chapter focuses on how the treating clinician addresses the psychological and social implication for people who live with seizures. Specific attention is paid towards co-morbid depression and suicide, as well as stigma associated with epilepsy, and the vocational and lifestyle implications of having seizures.

Psychological Aspects

Many clinicians underestimate the psychological impact that epilepsy may have on a patient. Even the diagnosis of a seizure disorder itself can have a significant effect on mood and interpersonal relationships. All patients with epilepsy should have regular reviews, and be specifically assessed for signs of depression from the early stages of diagnosis.

Depression

Although depression is a common co-morbid disease amongst patients with epilepsy, it is likely to be under-diagnosed, as it is not always routinely assessed in all neurology clinics.

Up to 55% of patients with uncontrolled epilepsy suffer from depression, and would fulfil the formal DSM-IV criteria. [1,2] However, even patients with well-controlled seizures have higher rates of depression than the general population. In addition, patients with epilepsy are four times more likely to be hospitalised for depression. [3]

The type of seizure that the person is affected by is another variable that affects mental health. Patients with complex partial seizures (CPS), in particular those with involvement of limbic structures, are more likely to suffer from depressive and anxiety symptoms than those with primary generalised epilepsy (PGE). [4] This adds weight to the argument that it is not just the psychological reaction to having seizures that leads to depression, but rather that there are likely neurobiochemical pathways that are implicated also.

It is also important to note that although depressive disorders can present as unipolar, bipolar or dysthymic disorders, patients with epilepsy often present with an atypical depression. [5] This may make symptoms unrecognisable for longer periods of times, stressing the importance of active surveillance. Clinical vigilance is required to pick up seemingly subtle symptoms. All patients with epilepsy should have regular reviews, and be assessed for signs of depression, as well as specifically questioned about their mood. Attention should be closely paid for need for formal referral to a psychologist or psychiatrist.

Fast and efficient screening tools have been developed to help with such assessments, such as the neurological disorders depression inventory for epilepsy (NDDI-E). [6] This tool specifically uses items to identify symptoms of depression that do not overlap with common adverse effects of antiepileptic drugs and common co-morbid cognitive deficits, which could be misinterpreted as signs of depression (e.g. fatigue, loss of appetite). Such tools are simple to use, with reliable sensitivity and specificity for the diagnosis of major depression in patients with epilepsy, to help facilitate prompt recognition.

The treating clinician must be aware of, and recognise the psychiatric effects of antiepileptic drugs (AEDs). For example, topiramate and levetiracetam are commonly used AEDs, but are known to potentiate mood disturbances, and even psychosis in severe cases. In patients with co-morbid psychiatric illness, such agents should generally be avoided, or used very cautiously if other treatment options have been exhausted. Other medications, such as sodium valproate, can have an additional benefit apart from its antiepileptic effect, due to its mood-stabilising properties. One should also be aware of this medication masking an underlying affective disorder, especially if consideration is being given to withdrawing the drug.

Once recognised, treatment of depression in the patient with seizures should be commenced promptly. Both pharmacological and non-pharmacological approaches are important. There is often hesitance in starting antidepressant medications due to concerns about drug interactions and additional side effects. [7] In particular, fears of lowering seizure threshold are often a major barrier to prescribing antidepressant drugs. Over 50% of primary care physicians identify this latter factor as a reason for not treating depression in patients with epilepsy. [7] In general, this effect is often very overestimated, and is most likely overshadowed by the risks of leaving the patient's depression untreated. Also, first line medications for depression such as the selective serotonin reuptake inhibitors (SSRIs) are generally quite safe in this regard, and should be considered as initial therapy. [5]

As mentioned, non-pharmacological treatments such as cognitive behavioural therapy are also an important adjunct, or even alternate option to the patient with mild depression who may be reluctant to taking any further medications.

Finally, the surgical option of vagal nerve stimulation may provide some benefit for both seizure control and improvement in mood. This therapeutic option should, however, be reserved for particularly refractory cases of epilepsy and depression, and the exact effectiveness of this intervention is unclear at this stage.

Suicide

Overall, suicide rates are around tripled in patients with epilepsy as compared with the background population. Although in part this is due to psychiatric, demographic, and socioeconomic factors, individuals with epilepsy are still at higher risk of suicide when these factors are taken into account. [8] Those with newly diagnosed epilepsy are particularly vulnerable and require special attention, as their risk is highest in the first six months after diagnosis. However, risk remains elevated throughout life, even in those with good seizure control. Those with a pre-existing history of psychiatric disease are at even greater risk

More recently, several antiepileptic drugs (AEDs) have been implicated in causing higher rates of suicidal thoughts and action. [1] In 2008 the Food and Drug Administration (FDA) raised concerns of an increased risk of suicidal thoughts and behaviour in patients taking AEDs.

This report was based on comparing treatment and placebo groups in various add-on studies. [9] Overall, the topic still remains quite contentious, and clear evidence for AEDs significantly increasing risk of suicide is still lacking.

The risks associated with uncontrolled seizures are much more likely to outweigh any increased risk of AED associated suicide risk, even in patients with co-morbid psychiatric disease. Such findings, however, do further stress the importance of routinely assessing mood in any patient with seizures, but perhaps with additional attention if they are starting a new AED.

Social Aspects

People with seizures may require social adjustments to be made after their diagnosis such that social and/or vocational rehabilitation may be needed. Co-morbid psychiatric illness described above may also contribute to these issues. Epilepsy requires a multidisciplinary psychosocial approach in dealing with this from the early stages of each patient's diagnosis and management, as this will shape the way the disease is impacted on in the future. [10]

Stigma

Unfortunately, compared with other disease, epilepsy is a condition that often has relatively little awareness amongst the general community. This is a striking fact given that it is such a common condition, affecting around one percent of the global population. There is also a lack of quantitative information on the exact psychosocial impact and socioeconomic consequences specific to patients with epilepsy, as well as their families. [11] However, it is quite clear that social ignorance and discrimination against people living with epilepsy is often a major barrier to integration with society. [12] At least 25% of adults with epilepsy describe social stigma as a result of their condition. [13] Stigma has been associated with seizures for thousands of years, sadly remaining ever present today, leading to social isolation and negative educational and occupational consequences.

The stigma surrounding this disease is seen in both developed and developing countries, but with significant variation from country to country, based on cultural differences and historical understandings. [14] It is certainly recognised as a major factor that contributes to the burden associated with epilepsy overall, but this burden can be enormous, and usually underestimated. It is often the most significant issue identified by the person with epilepsy in daily life, rather than the severity or frequency of seizures themselves. It is this latter aspect, however, which tends to receive the majority of attention in the clinical setting. This emphasises the point that the proper treatment of epilepsy should not just focus on seizure control, but rather be about minimising the impact of this chronic disease on the patient's psychosocial wellbeing, of which seizure control is just one aspect.

Even the words that the medical profession and general public use to describe epilepsy influences our perceptions and social stigma attached to the condition, with studies showing that the term 'epileptic' has a far greater negative connotation and prejudice associated with it than the term 'people with epilepsy'. [15] Hence, the latter term is preferred, as it does not define the patient as merely a subject of their condition.

Reducing this stigma and its impact on patients is crucial to improving their quality of life. Social support and epilepsy foundations can play an invaluable role in bridging this gap, as reducing stigma and raising awareness with tailored educational campaigns should be a major focus of such support groups. [16] It is essential for the treating clinician to be aware of laws that protect discrimination against their patients and their civil, educational and employment rights. All patients should have access to counselling services and social workers.

Driving

Even if a person has very infrequent seizures, it only takes a momentary lapse in consciousness whilst driving for potentially devastating consequences. To be instructed not to drive, however, is likely to impose significant restrictions on a person's lifestyle, and possibly occupation. It can be a difficult task for the treating clinician to put such limitations on their patients. In countries such as Australia, driver licensing authority place a great amount of this responsibility onto the treating doctor. [17] This, however, can potentially cause a conflict between the clinician's medical and legal responsibilities, with a main concern of causing damage to the doctor-patient relationship.

There are guidelines that can be used to help make the decision regarding a patient's fitness to drive. Laws and regulations regarding driving and epilepsy vary widely between different countries, and even between states in countries such as the United States. [18, 19] In general, guidelines suggest a seizure-free period between 1-2 years before passing a person as fit to drive, but some countries permit shortening of this period on the recommendation by an experienced neurologist that seizure control is adequate. [20] Such instances that would permit driving sooner would be where a clearly identifiable and reversible trigger for a seizure is found, such as an acute febrile illness, when which appropriately corrected should return the patient back to their baseline seizure threshold and control. Another such instance regards patients that have seizures exclusively in sleep, where episodes during wakefulness and thus driving are far less likely to occur. Holding a commercial licence to drive requires a much longer seizure-free period, with much greater restrictions.

There is growing evidence that the electroencephalogram (EEG) can be utilised to help guide a patient's fitness to drive. Around the world, including Australia [21] and Norway [22], around 39% of neurologists use EEG when making this assessment. In the United Kingdom, if a license has been lost because of seizures, it will not be reinstated if there is generalized spike-wave activity in the EEG. Although there is inconsistency in the current literature as to whether the routine EEG can be used to risk stratify patients, a more prolonged day recording may better predict the likelihood of two-year seizure relapse. [23] Thus, this tool has the potential to minimise the risk of seizure-related motor vehicle accidents, [24] and although it has not yet been widely adopted, it is currently used by some major tertiary centres in making driving assessments.

Vocational

Most people with epilepsy can work normally, and a good general rule is that if fit to drive they are safe to work in most circumstances. A major problem for patients with seizures is unpredictability of the next seizure. Some patients have exclusively nocturnal seizures, and this is less of an issue, as also discussed above regarding driving. It is important to balance the risk of subsequent seizure with the psychosocial implications of placing restrictions on the patient's work and lifestyle. Similar to driving restriction, however, patients may need to be discouraged from certain activities in work and their social lives, which place them at increased risk of injury or death. These include working from heights or operating heavy machinery. If power tools are to be used, supervision may be needed, with the use of safety devices such as automatic shut-off switches recommended.

Poor seizure control is one reason for difficulty with employment amongst people with epilepsy. Psychiatric co-morbidity, as described previously, is another reason that inhibits people from being able to enter the workplace. However, even with these factors corrected, rates of unemployment are higher in people with epilepsy that are capable of working. Laws are present in most countries to protect individuals with disabilities from workplace discrimination. Unfortunately, these laws are frequency circumvented due to the subjective nature of hiring and retention of employees. The degree of social avoidance regarding epilepsy is higher than that of other conditions, including other neurological conditions such as multiple sclerosis. [25]

Individual attitudes are also an important factor in influencing employment status. Fear of workplace discrimination is one of the strongest factors that is negatively associated with employment in people with epilepsy. [26] Unfortunately such fears are often a reality, with high rates of allegations of workplace discrimination regarding hiring, as well as post-hire issues such as promotion and termination, disciplinary actions and harassment. [27]

Research has shown that much of the avoidant behaviour displayed by co-workers in the workplace stems from worry of a sudden, unpredictable event as well as their discomfort and fears in providing necessary first-aid should a seizure occur. [25] Thus, education of the patient's workplace, or school, is a productive and effective way to increase understanding and minimise stigma associated with seizures, [28] given that these are the environments from which much of the patient's perception of stigma are derived from. [29]

Such vocational rehabilitation programs have shown encouraging results with enhancing employment rates and work productivity, as well as work satisfaction. Seizure action plans are a useful part of this process, such that misconceptions are demystified for those surrounding people living with epilepsy in their day-to-day lives.

Lifestyle

As with driving and work restrictions such as operating heavy machinery, a certain degree of caution must also be applied to other daily activities outside of work. Common sense is really the most important part in guiding any restrictions or modifications that are required, such that any situation where an unexpected loss of consciousness would pose an immediate danger to the person should be avoided. Prevention of drowning is an exemplar of this, as the risk of drowning in people with epilepsy is 15- to 19-fold higher compared with the general population. [30] If there is any ongoing risk of seizure recurrence, swimming or bathing require supervision, and showers should be advised for patients that live alone. It is always prudent for the treating clinician to reiterate and advise their patients on such prevention strategies.

Conclusion

To date, the primary focus of epilepsy research has regarded itself with medical therapies. However, to provide comprehensive, or perhaps even the most basic of care for the patient with epilepsy, efforts must also address the psychosocial aspects, as these are the issues that greatly impact on quality of life. Psychiatric disease and epilepsy have a two-directional relationship, as those with major depression have a higher frequency of epilepsy, and those with epilepsy are more susceptible to depressive and anxiety disorders.

Addressing concurrent depressive symptoms, stigma and social support is paramount, and should be part of routine care. Patients should have access to written and visual information, counselling services, information about voluntary organisations and epilepsy specialist nurses. The expertise of multidisciplinary teams is required to manage more complicated cases of epilepsy and should include neuropsychology, neuropsychiatry and social work.

References

AUSTROADS, Commission ANRT. *Assessing fitness to drive for commercial and private vehicle drivers*. 2006. http://www.austroads.com.au/cms/AFTD%20web%20Aug%202006.pdf

Bagary M. Epilepsy, antiepileptic drugs and suicidality. *Curr. Opin. Neurol.* 2011;24(2): 177-182.

Bautista RED, Wludyka P. Factors associated with employment in epilepsy patients. *Epilepsy Behav.* 2007;10(1):89-95.

Bell GS, Gaitatzis A, Bell CL, Johnson AL, Sander JW. Drowning in people with epilepsy: how great is the risk? *Neurology.* 2008;71(8):578-582.

Beran RG, Ainley LAE, Beran ME. Opinions, attitudes and practices of Australian neurologists with regard to epilepsy and driving. *Intern Med J.* 2007;37(4):251-257.

Brodtkorb E, Bråthen G, Bovim G, Helde G. [Disagreement about epilepsy and driving]. *Tidsskr. Nor. Laegeforen.* 2004;124(8):1100-1102.

Christensen J, Vestergaard M, Mortensen PB, Sidenius P, Agerbo E. Epilepsy and risk of suicide: a population-based case-control study. *Lancet Neurol.* 2007;6(8):693-698.

Cotterman-Hart S. Depression in epilepsy: why aren't we treating? *Epilepsy Behav.* 2010;19(3):419-421.

de Boer HM. Epilepsy stigma: moving from a global problem to global solutions. *Seizure.* 2010;19(10):630-636.

Fernandes PT, de Barros NF, Li LM. Stop saying epileptic. *Epilepsia.* 2009;50(5):1280-1283.

Fernandes PT, Snape DA, Beran RG, Jacoby A. Epilepsy stigma: What do we know and where next? *Epilepsy Behav.* 2011.

Fisher R, Parsonage M, Beaussart M. Epilepsy and driving: an international perspective. *Epilepsia.* 1994.

Fowle AJ, Binnie CD. Uses and abuses of the EEG in epilepsy. *Epilepsia.* 2000;41 Suppl 3:S10-8.

French JA, Pedley TA. Clinical practice. Initial management of epilepsy. *N. Engl. J. Med.* 2008;359(2):166-176.

Gilliam FG, Barry JJ, Hermann BP, et al. Rapid detection of major depression in epilepsy: a multicentre study. *Lancet Neurol.* 2006;5(5):399-405.

Gülpek D, Bolat E, Mete L, Arici S, Celebisoy M. Psychiatric comorbidity, quality of life and social support in epileptic patients. *Nord J Psychiatry.* 2011.

Hackett ML, Glozier NS, Martiniuk AL, Jan S, Anderson CS. Sydney epilepsy incidence study to measure illness consequences: the SESIMIC observational epilepsy study protocol. *BMC Neurol.* 2011;11:3.

Harden CL, Kossoy A, Vera S, Nikolov B. Reaction to epilepsy in the workplace. *Epilepsia.* 2004;45(9):1134-1140.

Indaco A, Carrieri PB, Nappi C, Gentile S, Striano S. Interictal depression in epilepsy. *Epilepsy Res.* 1992;12(1):45-50.

Kamel JT, Christensen B, Odell MS, D'Souza WJ, Cook MJ. Evaluating the use of prolonged video-EEG monitoring to assess future seizure risk and fitness to drive. *Epilepsy Behav.* 2010;19(4):608-611.

Kanner AM, Nieto JC. Depressive disorders in epilepsy. *Neurology*. 1999;53(5 Suppl 2): S26-32.

Karouni M, Arulthas S, Larsson PG, et al. Psychiatric comorbidity in patients with epilepsy: a population-based study. *Eur. J. Clin. Pharmacol.* 2010;66(11):1151-1160.

Krumholz A. Driving and epilepsy: a historical perspective and review of current regulations. *Epilepsia*. 1994;35(3):668-674.

Kubota H. [Social support for people with epilepsy]. *Brain Nerve*. 2011;63(4):401-409..Bandstra NF, Camfield CS, Camfield PR. Stigma of epilepsy. *Can J Neurol Sci.* 2008;35(4):436-440.

Loring DW, Hermann BP, Cohen MJ. Neuropsychological advocacy and epilepsy. *Clin Neuropsychol.* 2010;24(3):417-428.

Mendez MF, Cummings JL, Benson DF. Depression in epilepsy. Significance and phenomenology. *Arch. Neurol.* 1986;43(8):766-770.

Smith G, Ferguson PL, Saunders LL, et al. Psychosocial factors associated with stigma in adults with epilepsy. *Epilepsy Behav*. 2009;16(3):484-490.

Somerville ER, Black AB, Dunne JW. Driving to distraction--certification of fitness to drive with epilepsy. *Med. J. Aust.* 2010;192(6):342-344.

West MD, Dye AN, McMahon BT. Epilepsy and workplace discrimination: population characteristics and trends. *Epilepsy and Behavior*. 2006;9(1):101-105.

In: Seizures and Anti-Epileptic Drugs
Editors: Willard Hosten and Aleph Burtsev
ISBN: 978-1-62100-255-0

Chapter X

Pharmacokinetic Interactions between Antiepileptic Drugs and Oral Contraceptives and Clinical Consequences

Anne Sabers*
The Epilepsy Clinic, Department of Neurology, University State Hospital, Rigshospitalet, Copenhagen, Denmark

Abstract

Pharmacokinetics of antiepileptic drugs (AED's) and oral contraceptives (OC's) can interact bi-directionally. AED's have a potential influence on the effect of OC's and pose thereby a risk of un-intended pregnancy as well as OC's may decrease the effect of some AED's and increase the risk of seizure deterioration. The consequences are of major concern. Contraceptive failure may be disastrous for most women but is critical for women who are taking AED's because of the teratogenetic potential of the AED's. In addition, AED failure can seriously influence on many psychosocial aspects of the patient's life.

The magnitude of the drug-drug interactions shows in general wide inter-individual variability and the change in the elimination rate is often unpredictable and can be influenced by a number of co-variants. Change in OC use should therefore be assisted by AED monitoring and adequate dose adjustment whenever possible and AED's without pharmacokinetic interaction potentials may be considered as drug of first choices for women who use OC's.

* E-mail: anne.sabers@rh.regionh.dk, a@sabers.dk.

Introduction

Epilepsy is a common neurological disorder that affects 0.4–0.8% of the population [1]. With the increasing use of antiepileptic drugs (AED's) for indications other than epilepsy [2], the proportion of women with a childbearing potential that take AED's is substantial. Oral contraceptives (OC's) are prescribed for approximately 20 % of fertile women with epilepsy depending on cultural and religious considerations [3;4] and co-administration of AED's and OC's is therefore a common clinical situation that calls for specific considerations of possible drugs interactions.

Combined OC's and AED's can interact bi-directionally. The main consequences of these pharmacokinetic interactions are risks of therapeutic failures of both treatments. Contraceptive failure with the result of un-intended pregnancy is disastrous situation for most women but is of even higher critical concern for women who are taking AED's because of the teratogenetic potential of the drugs. Numerous studies have demonstrated that there is a two to three fold increased risk of major congenital malformations following fetal exposure of certain AED's [5]. The risk of AED failure is also of major concern as seizure relapse or increased seizure frequency in some situations can be life threatening or seriously affect many psychosocial aspects of the patient's life.

A surprising number of physicians do not have adequate knowledge about potential interactions between AED's and OC's [6]. Approximately 50 % of women with epilepsy who take OC's indicate that they have never received information about this specific issue [7-9]. However, it has also been shown that these women not always recall being given information on contraception, which highlights the need for regular repetition of this type of information [10].

Treating women with epilepsy of fertile age includes systematic, ongoing and accurate counseling on optimal choice of contraception. The widely available range of AED's stresses the importance of being familiar with the various properties of the drugs and to achieve a better understanding of the drug-drug interactions.

The Effect AED's on the Pharmcokinetics of Combined OC's

The most widely used OC's is combined steroid formulations containing an estrogen (usually ethinylestradiol) and a progestin compound. A potential for interaction between AED's and OC's was first suggested in the early 1970's, about 10 years after the introduction of combined steroid OC's. A higher incidence of breakthrough bleeding and contraceptive failure among women with epilepsy was observed and correlated with the time at which the ethinylestradiol fraction of the OC's was decreased from 50–100 μg to less than 50 μg to diminish the risk of thromboembolic side effects. Most modern combined OC preparations contain 20–35 μg of ethinylestradiol and less than 1 mg of progestin. Ethinylestradiol undergoes significant first pass metabolism in the gut by sulphation and in the liver by glucuronidation and hydroxylation. Most of the estrogen compound is hydroxylated to inactive metabolites, catalyzed by the hepatic cytochrome P450 (CYP) 3A4. Metabolites undergo conjugation and enterohepatic recirculation, resulting in re-absorption of active ethinylestradiol.

Most AED's available in the 1970–1980's; carbamazepine [11], phenobarbital [12], and phenytoin [13] induce the hepatic CYP3A4 isoenzyme and therefore can accelerate hepatic elimination of OC's, thus increasing the risk of contraceptive failure. Also some of the second generation AED's; felbamate [14], oxcarbazepine [15], and topiramate [16] induce subtypes of the P450 system and can reduce the OC efficacy. The new AED compound eslicarbazepine acetate shares some of the chemical structures of carbamazepine and oxcarbazepine but does not share structures responsible for the enzyme induction [17]. However, eslicarbazepine acetate can decrease the hormonal components of OC in a minor way that may be clinical relevant for some patients [18].

The extent of enzyme induction seems to be correlated with the dose of the drug, but this is difficult to quantify and pose wide inter-individually variation as genetic and environmental factors also influence hepatic isoenzyme expression [19]. This can be exemplified by topiramate that in monotherapy at dosages less than 200 mg not significantly affect the clinical efficacy of combined OC's containing a moderate dosage of ethinylestradiol (35 μg)[20]. Thus, OC's containing 35 μg ethinylestradiol might remain sufficiently active in women receiving low dose topiramate monotherapy whereas for all other enzyme inducing AED's is it generally recommended that women who are taking these AED's use high-dose OC's (estrogen compound dosage of at least 50 μg) in combination with barrier methods of contraception [21]. Alternatively, it has also been suggested that women using AED's with a enzyme inducing potential should use combined OC's that contain a progestin dosage well above that needed to inhibit ovulation and that they take the contraceptive continuously without a pill-free interval [22]. However, there are no published data to support the efficacy of this strategy.

Even though the potential for interaction between enzyme-inducing AED's and OC's has been known for many years, widespread incorporation of this information into everyday practice is still lacking. In the study by Shorvon et al. (2002)[23] it was reported that of 2000 women taking enzyme-inducing AED's, more than 50 % were taking OC's with an estrogen content less than 50 μg. Considering that more than 50 % of pregnancies in the population with epilepsy are unplanned, partly because of contraceptive failure [24], this is a matter of considerable concern.

Among the non-enzyme inducting AED's available data suggest that neither valproate [25], gabapentin [26], levetiracetam [27], tiagabine [28], vigabatrin [29], zonisamide [30], rufinamide [31], nor lacosamide [17] influence the metabolism of OC's and these AED's can therefore be administrated without risk of contraceptive failure. Lamotrigine, however, may have a modest effect of the plasma level of the levonorgestrel compound of OC's [32] but the ethinylestradiol compound is affected and is thereby probably not clinically relevant. This is in agreement with the former study by Holdich et al. (1991), who found no effect of lamotrigine on the elimination of OC's [33]. When interpreting these data it is important to consider that the women in these studies were taking moderate-dose OC's that contained 35 μg ethinylestradiol plus 150 μg levonorgestrel. Ovulation may not be suppressed in women who use low-dose OC's that contain less than 30 μg ethinylestradiol and 75 μg progestin. Therefore, midcycle bleeding should always alert the physician and the patient to the risk of contraceptive failure.

Few data about possible interactions between AED's and progestin-only pills (Mini-pills) are available. Enzyme-inducing AED's increases the metabolism of progestins as well as estrogens and progestin-only OC's containing less than 0.5 mg progestin should probably not be regarded as effective. There are no data of what dose of progestin that is needed for emergency contraception following unprotected intercourse in women who use enzyme-inducing AED's but current guidelines generally recommended approximately the double dose of progestin; 1.5 mg levonorgestrel as soon as possible and followed by 0.75 mg 12 hours after.

The Effect of Combined OC's on the Pharmacokinetics of AED's

Estrogen-containing OC's induce the hepatic enzyme uridine 5'-diphosphate-glucuronosyltransferase 1A4 (UGT1A4), an isoenzyme of the UGT family of enzymes. Thus, the metabolism of drugs that are eliminated by glucuronic acid conjugation catalyzed by this enzyme might be increased in women taking OC's. Among AED's, this metabolic pathway has been studied most intensively for lamotrigine but also valproate, oxcarbazepine and eslicarbazepine acetat are metabolized by glucuronic acid conjugation. Lamotrigine is primary glucuronidated and the elimination is accelerated more that 50 % by co-treatment with combined OC's [32;34-39] . The effect of OC on lamotrigine metabolism appears to be attributed the estrogen rather than the progestin component of the contraceptives [40]. The urine excretion of the *N*-2-glucuronide metabolite / lamotrigine ratio was significantly higher in women who were taking combined OC's than in women who did not, indicating that the pharmacokinetic mechanism of the drug interaction was an alteration of metabolic glucuronidation processes [35;38]. It has also been found that there is considerable inter-individual variability in the extent of the pharmacokinetic alterations, probably due to both genetic and extrinsic factors, such as co-administration of other AED's. For example, Tomson et al. (2006) demonstrated that the OC-induced increase in lamotrigine metabolism was almost eliminated when valproate, another glucuronidated AED, was co-administered [41]. The effect of OC's on the elimination of lamotrigine is linear and acute and the plasma level of lamotrigine reach de-induced levels in the end of the "pill-free" week [32;34;42][38]. The progestin only component of OC's (Mini-pills) does not seem to affect the metabolism of lamotrigine [40].

The other AED's that are partially or fully eliminated by glucuronidation may have a similar interaction with combined OC's. One study reported that plasma concentrations of valproate were significantly lower with than without concomitant administration of combined OC's but that the difference was less pronounced than that for a parallel lamotrigine-treatment group [43]. Another group reported that the plasma clearance of the unbound fraction of valproate was almost doubled during concomitant use of OC [44]. Concerning oxcarbazepine, in particular the pharmacologically active monohydroxy derivate of oxcarbazepine (MHD) is eliminated mainly by glucuronidation, but the clinical relevance of a potential OC-MHD interaction needs further evaluation. The same seems to be the case for eslicarbazepine acetate.

The potential consequences of the increased elimination processes of these glucuronidated AED's by OC are highly clinically relevant and serve to underscore the importance of monitoring the drug plasma levels of these drugs following initiation or discontinuation of OC's. A drop in plasma levels of the drugs following initiation of OC's may lead to increased seizure activity [36] and on the contrary side effects may occur following OC discontinuation of dosages are not adjusted. Overdose symptoms that can occur even after discontinuation of the OC in the "pill-free" week, and be disregarded as menstruation-related headache, fatigue, and dizziness if not properly interpreted. When women prepare to discontinue OC's in order to become pregnant, the dosage of the AED should be adjusted to avoid unnecessarily high drug exposure to the fetus at time of conception. Due to this problem it has also been suggested that up-titration of lamotrigine dosage should not occur during the "pill-free week" in order to avoid potential titration-related tolerability problems [32]. Similar, blood sampling for lamotrigine may need to be standardized according to the OC cycles. Estrogen containing OC's are frequently used as hormonal replacement therapy for menopausal symptoms. Lamotrigine levels are decreased in postmenopausal women who use estrogen hormonal therapy in the same way as in patients using the tablets for contraception [45].

Conclusion

Interactions between AED's and OC's may have serious clinical consequences. It is therefore recommended that change in OC use is assisted by AED monitoring and adequate dose adjustment whenever possible as well as the educational level about these interactions should be highlighted. However, the information is notoriously hard to distribute and consolidate both among physicians and patients and AED's without a drug-drug interaction potential may therefore be preferable treatment choices for women with epilepsy in fertile age.

References

[1] Wallace H, Shorvon S, Tallis R: Age-specific incidence and prevalence rates of treated epilepsy in an unselected population of 2,052,922 and age-specific fertility rates of women with epilepsy. *Lancet* 1998;352:1970-1973.

[2] Spina E, Perugi G: Antiepileptic drugs: indications other than epilepsy. *Epileptic* Disord 2004;6:57-75.

[3] Shorvon SD, Tallis RC, Wallace HK: Antiepileptic drugs: coprescription of proconvulsant drugs and oral contraceptives: a national study of antiepileptic drug prescribing practice. *J Neurol Neurosurg Psychiatry* 2002;72:114-115.

[4] Cibula D: Women's contraceptive practices and sexual behaviour in Europe. *Eur J Contracept Reprod Health Care* 2008;13:362-375.

[5] Harden CL, Meador KJ, Pennell PB, Hauser WA, Gronseth GS, French JA, Wiebe S, Thurman D, Koppel BS, Kaplan PW, Robinson JN, Hopp J, Ting TY, Gidal B, Hovinga CA, Wilner AN, Vazquez B, Holmes L, Krumholz A, Finnell R, Hirtz D, Le GC:

Management issues for women with epilepsy-Focus on pregnancy (an evidence-based review): II. Teratogenesis and perinatal outcomes: Report of the Quality Standards Subcommittee and Therapeutics and Technology Subcommittee of the American Academy of Neurology and the American Epilepsy Society. *Epilepsia* 2009;50: 1237-1246.

[6] Shorvon SD, Tallis RC, Wallace HK: Antiepileptic drugs: coprescription of proconvulsant drugs and oral contraceptives: a national study of antiepileptic drug prescribing practice. *J Neurol Neurosurg Psychiatry* 2002;72:114-115.

[7] Long L, Montouris G: Knowledge of women's issues and epilepsy (KOWIE-II): a survey of health care professionals. *Epilepsy Behav* 2005;6:90-93.

[8] Kampman MT, Johansen SV, Stenvold H, Acharya G: Management of women with epilepsy: Are guidelines being followed? Results from case-note reviews and a patient questionnaire. *Epilepsia* 2005;46:1286-1292.

[9] Pack AM, Davis AR, Kritzer J, Yoon A, Camus A: Antiepileptic drugs: are women aware of interactions with oral contraceptives and potential teratogenicity? *Epilepsy Behav* 2009;14:640-644.

[10] Bell GS, Nashef L, Kendall S, Solomon J, Poole K, Johnson AL, Moran NF, McCarthy M, McCormick D, Shorvon SD, Sander JW: Information recalled by women taking anti-epileptic drugs for epilepsy: a questionnaire study. *Epilepsy Res* 2002;52:139-146.

[11] Crawford P, Chadwick DJ, Martin C, Tjia J, Back DJ, Orme M: The interaction of phenytoin and carbamazepine with combined oral contraceptive steroids. *Br J Clin Pharmacol* 1990;30:892-896.

[12] Back DJ, Orme ML: Pharmacokinetic drug interactions with oral contraceptives. *Clin Pharmacokinet* 1990;18:472-484.

[13] Crawford P, Chadwick DJ, Martin C, Tjia J, Back DJ, Orme M: The interaction of phenytoin and carbamazepine with combined oral contraceptive steroids. *Br J Clin Pharmacol* 1990;30:892-896.

[14] Saano V, Glue P, Banfield CR, Reidenberg P, Colucci RD, Meehan JW, Haring P, Radwanski E, Nomeir A, Lin CC,: Effects of felbamate on the pharmacokinetics of a low-dose combination oral contraceptive. *Clin Pharmacol Ther* 1995;58:523-531.

[15] Fattore C, Cipolla G, Gatti G, Limido GL, Sturm Y, Bernasconi C, Perucca E: Induction of ethinylestradiol and levonorgestrel metabolism by oxcarbazepine in healthy women. *Epilepsia* 1999;40:783-787.

[16] Rosenfeld WE, Doose DR, Walker SA, Nayak RK: Effect of topiramate on the pharmacokinetics of an oral contraceptive containing norethindrone and ethinyl estradiol in patients with epilepsy. *Epilepsia* 1997;38:317-323.

[17] Bialer M, Johannessen SI, Kupferberg HJ, Levy RH, Perucca E, Tomson T: Progress report on new antiepileptic drugs: a summary of the Eigth Eilat Conference (EILAT VIII). *Epilepsy Res* 2007;73:1-52.

[18] Almeida L, Soares-da-Silva P: Eslicarbazepine acetate (BIA 2-093). *Neurotherapeutics* 2007;4:88-96.

[19] Tomson T, Svensson JO, Hilton-Brown P: Relationship of intraindividual dose to plasma concentration of carbamazepine: indication of dose-dependent induction of metabolism. *Ther Drug Monit* 1989;11:533-539.

[20] Doose DR, Wang SS, Padmanabhan M, Schwabe S, Jacobs D, Bialer M: Effect of topiramate or carbamazepine on the pharmacokinetics of an oral contraceptive

containing norethindrone and ethinyl estradiol in healthy obese and nonobese female subjects. *Epilepsia* 2003;44:540-549.

[21] Practice parameter: management issues for women with epilepsy (summary statement). Report of the Quality Standards Subcommittee of the American Academy of Neurology: *Neurology* 1998;51:944-948.

[22] Schwenkhagen AM, Stodieck SR: Which contraception for women with epilepsy? *Seizure* 2008;17:145-150.

[23] Shorvon SD, Tallis RC, Wallace HK: Antiepileptic drugs: coprescription of proconvulsant drugs and oral contraceptives: a national study of antiepileptic drug prescribing practice. *J Neurol Neurosurg Psychiatry* 2002;72:114-115.

[24] Fairgrieve SD, Jackson M, Jonas P, Walshaw D, White K, Montgomery TL, Burn J, Lynch SA: Population based, prospective study of the care of women with epilepsy in pregnancy. *BMJ* 2000;321:674-675.

[25] Crawford P, Chadwick D, Cleland P, Tjia J, Cowie A, Back DJ, Orme ML: The lack of effect of sodium valproate on the pharmacokinetics of oral contraceptive steroids. *Contraception* 1986;33:23-29.

[26] Eldon MA, Underwood BA, Randinitis EJ, Sedman AJ: Gabapentin does not interact with a contraceptive regimen of norethindrone acetate and ethinyl estradiol. *Neurology* 1998;50:1146-1148.

[27] Ragueneau-Majlessi I, Levy RH, Janik F: Levetiracetam does not alter the pharmacokinetics of an oral contraceptive in healthy women. *Epilepsia* 2002;43: 697-702.

[28] Mengel HB, Houston A, Back D.J: An evaluation of the interaction between tiagabine and oral contraceptives in female volunteers. *Journal of Pharmacology and Medicine* 1994;4:141-150.

[29] Bartoli A, Gatti G, Cipolla G, Barzaghi N, Veliz G, Fattore C, Mumford J, Perucca E: A double-blind, placebo-controlled study on the effect of vigabatrin on in vivo parameters of hepatic microsomal enzyme induction and on the kinetics of steroid oral contraceptives in healthy female volunteers. *Epilepsia* 1997;38:702-707.

[30] Griffith SG, Dai Y: Effect of zonisamide on the pharmacokinetics and pharmacodynamics of a combination ethinyl estradiol-norethindrone oral contraceptive in healthy women. *Clin Ther* 2004;26:2056-2065.

[31] Perucca E, Cloyd J, Critchley D, Fuseau E: Rufinamide: clinical pharmacokinetics and concentration-response relationships in patients with epilepsy. *Epilepsia* 2008;49: 1123-1141.

[32] Sidhu J, Job S, Singh S, Philipson R: The pharmacokinetic and pharmacodynamic consequences of the co-administration of lamotrigine and a combined oral contraceptive in healthy female subjects. *Br J Clin Pharmacol* 2006;61:191-199.

[33] Holdich T, Whiteman P, Orme M, Back D, Ward S: Effect of lamotrigine on the pharmacology of the combined oral contraceptive pill. *Epilepsia* 1991;32:96.

[34] Contin M, Albani F, Ambrosetto G, Avoni P, Bisulli F, Riva R, Tinuper P, Baruzzi A: Variation in lamotrigine plasma concentrations with hormonal contraceptive monthly cycles in patients with epilepsy. *Epilepsia* 2006;47:1573-1575.

[35] Ohman I, Luef G, Tomson T: Effects of pregnancy and contraception on lamotrigine disposition: new insights through analysis of lamotrigine metabolites. *Seizure* 2008;17:199-202.

[36] Sabers A, Buchholt JM, Uldall P, Hansen EL: Lamotrigine plasma levels reduced by oral contraceptives. *Epilepsy Res* 2001;47:151-154.
[37] Sabers A, Ohman I, Christensen J, Tomson T: Oral contraceptives reduce lamotrigine plasma levels. *Neurology* 2003;61:570-571.
[38] Christensen J, Petrenaite V, Atterman J, Sidenius P, Ohman I, Tomson T, Sabers A: Oral contraceptives induce lamotrigine metabolism: evidence from a double-blind, placebo-controlled trial. *Epilepsia* 2007;48:484-489.
[39] Wegner I, Edelbroek PM, Bulk S, Lindhout D: Lamotrigine kinetics within the menstrual cycle, after menopause, and with oral contraceptives. *Neurology* 2009;73:1388-1393.
[40] Reimers A, Helde G, Brodtkorb E: Ethinyl estradiol, not progestogens, reduces lamotrigine serum concentrations. *Epilepsia* 2005;46:1414-1417.
[41] Tomson T, Luef G, Sabers A, Pittschieler S, Ohman I: Valproate effects on kinetics of lamotrigine in pregnancy and treatment with oral contraceptives. *Neurology* 2006;67:1297-1299.
[42] Wegner I, Edelbroek P, de Haan GJ, Lindhout D, Sander JW: Drug monitoring of lamotrigine and oxcarbazepine combination during pregnancy. E*pilepsia* 2010;51: 2500-2502.
[43] Herzog AG, Blum AS, Farina EL, Maestri XE, Newman J, Garcia E, Krishnamurthy KB, Hoch DB, Replansky S, Fowler KM, Smithson SD, Dworetzky BA, Bromfield EB: Valproate and lamotrigine level variation with menstrual cycle phase and oral contraceptive use. *Neurology* 2009;72:911-914.
[44] Galimberti CA, Mazzucchelli I, Arbasino C, Canevini MP, Fattore C, Perucca E: Increased apparent oral clearance of valproic acid during intake of combined contraceptive steroids in women with epilepsy. *Epilepsia* 2006;47:1569-1572.
[45] Harden CL, Herzog AG, Nikolov BG, Koppel BS, Christos PJ, Fowler K, Labar DR, Hauser WA: Hormone replacement therapy in women with epilepsy: a randomized, double-blind, placebo-controlled study. *Epilepsia* 2006;47:1447-1451.

Index

A

B

C

D

E

F

G

H

M

N

O

P

Q

R

S

T